REVENUE CYCLE MANAGEMENT

Don't Get Lost in the Financial Maze

By
Kem Tolliver, CMPE, CPC
Shawntea Moheiser, CMPE, CMOM

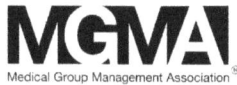

MGMA
Medical Group Management Association®

Medical Group Management Association© (MGMA©) publications are intended to provide current and accurate information and are designed to assist readers in becoming more familiar with the subject matter covered. Such publications are distributed with the understanding that MGMA does not render any legal, accounting, or other professional advice that may be construed as specifically applicable to an individual situation. No representations or warranties are made concerning the application of legal or other principles discussed by the authors to any specific factual situation, nor is any prediction made concerning how any particular judge, government official, or other person will interpret or apply such principles. Specific factual situations should be discussed with professional advisors.

Published By: MGMA

Production / Partner Publisher: EGZ Publications

Library of Congress Cataloging-in-Publication Data

Names: Tolliver, Kem (Kemberly), 1974- author. | Moheiser, Shawntea, 1984- author. | MGMA (Association), issuing body. Title: Revenue Cycle Management : Don't Get Lost in the Financial Maze / by Kem Tolliver, Shawntea Moheiser.
Description: Englewood, Colorado : MGMA, Medical Group Management Association, 2019. | Includes bibliographical references and index.
Identifiers: LCCN 2019035882 (print) | LCCN 2019035883 (ebook) | ISBN 9781568296777 (paperback) | ISBN 9781568296784 (ebook)
Subjects: MESH: Financial Management | Practice Management, Medical--economics | Fees, Medical | United States
Classification: LCC RA971.3 (print) | LCC RA971.3 (ebook) | NLM W 80 | DDC 362.1068/1--dc23
LC record available at https://lccn.loc.gov/2019035882   LC ebook record available at https://lccn.loc.gov/2019035883

Published in Centennial Colorado
by
the Medical Group Management Association

Printed in the United States of America 10 9 8 7 6 5 4 3 2 1

Dedication

To the giants we rub shoulders with
every day in our shared quest to
transform healthcare management.

Acknowledgments

~ Taya Moheiser~
Eleanor Roosevelt once said, "What is to give light must endure the burning."
Wow is this an excellent analogy for the book writing process!

Matt, thank you for feeding me, reminding me to take breaks, totally holding down the fort, uplifting my spirits, instilling confidence, and encouraging me to keep going when it felt it was too big a mountain to climb. Alyssa, thank you for the sporadic cuddles and of course the several hundred Rice Krispie's treats. To Stephen & Thomas, thank you for staying out of trouble for a bit so I didn't lose focus. To my dad and my sister, thank you so much for the planning and strategy tips, the venting sessions and, when needed, a good gut check.

To my mother-in-law for dragging me into healthcare over a decade ago, thank you for showing me where to find my passion. To all of the strong women in my family who showed me how to impact my community with wisdom, strength, and a velvet hammer. You remind me that, *"You don't make progress by standing on the sidelines, whimpering and complaining, you make progress by implementing ideas" – Shirley Chisolm.* Thank you to all of the friends who checked on me, under my rock, to send a little sunlight my way.

To my mom, Denise, there hasn't been a moment in my life you weren't my best supporter, greatest encourager and closest friend. Your giving spirit and thirst for knowledge are imprinted upon me and I am eternally grateful. You remind me to work hard, to do what's right, and to be true to myself. You are my rock.

I would be remiss if I didn't thank Craig and MGMA for entertaining this crazy idea of mine and Kem for your willingness to join in the crazy fun. Finally, thank you to the editors for tolerating a barrage of late night emails, instant messages and crying emojis. You're the real MVPs.

-Taya

~ **Kem Tolliver** ~
Life's most persistent and urgent question is,
"What are you doing for others?"
— Martin Luther King, Jr.

This book is dedicated to healthcare professionals and providers who master mazes each day for the healing of others. The persistence of my immigrant grandmothers and the strong women who mold me is equivalent to fortitude meets strength. They remind me that, *"Age wrinkles the body. Quitting wrinkles the soul." – Douglas MacArthur.*

Thank you to my husband Tyrone for everything, literally everything. Thank you to my children Tye and Sasha for giving me the two most important reasons to press on. I am grateful to my parents for allowing the hospital corridors to be my playground and the staff to become family while you made a living there. My heartfelt thanks to my sisters (genetic and chosen), brother, family, friends and clients for encouraging me throughout the book writing process. Pat, thank you for shouldering responsibility like the boss you are.

My sincerest appreciation to the physicians, managers, mentors, and colleagues who have sown individual seeds into me which have sparked my eternal flame for learning and educating others. Posthumous gratitude to Hector K. Collison, MD, FACC for my first job in healthcare and for nurturing my thirst for knowledge. I promise to keep, "Working hard and living good."

This book would not be possible without MGMA's promise of developing healthcare leaders and Taya's flashlight leading the way. *"One important key to success is self-confidence. An important key to self-confidence is preparation."* *–Arthur Ashe.* It is my prayer that you, the reader, will take the nuggets of information within this book to continue the cycle of healing.

-Kem

Contributors

Special gratitude is offered to those professionals who took the time to review, provide feedback, contribute and offer industry expertise during the writing of this book. The contributions of these individuals impacts the overall integrity of the book content and context of complex subject matter.

Larry Hefling Owner, ITS Strategic, LLC	**Jay Hodes** President, Colington Consulting	**Jenny Jacobsen,** JD Director of Cybersecurity, Silverstone
Stephen H. Kaufman, Esq. Partner, Wright, Constable & Skeen	**Luigi Leblanc,** MPH, CPHIT VP of Technology, Zane Networks	**Morgan Power** Director of Business Intelligence Think WholePerson Healthcare
Denise Walsh, CPC, CHSP Senior Coding Compliance Advisor, Medical Revenue Cycle Specialists	**Charletta Washington,** MHA President, Precision Healthcare Solutions	**Monica Wright,** CPC, CPMA Certified Professional Coder Certified Professional Medical Auditor

Contents

Contents

Preface

Dear Fellow Healthcare Colleagues,

Medical Group Management Association (MGMA) has given us the opportunity to develop and share this resource for revenue cycle management (RCM) with you. We envision this information to be useful and sharable with medical office front desk staff, call center staff, billing staff, coding staff, clinical staff, providers of healthcare and practice managers.

With fee for service almost in the rear-view mirror and pay for quality now a reality, it's time to transform the revenue cycle. Let's stave off our burnout as well as antiquated manual processes and instead embrace technology while leveraging quality payment programs. Our desire is to support your efforts in retaining and professionally developing yourself and your staff with the intended outcome of improved quality patient care.

The information in this book comprehensively describes and provides guidance on the management of key components within revenue cycle management in the medical office. This content is applicable to both individuals new to RCM, seasoned RCM professionals, as well as providers of care.

Given the vast amount of industry resources and information dedicated to hospitals and other large healthcare institutions, this book was designed to provide RCM strategies for private medical practices.

Within the book, there are essential strategies for orientation, continued development, and process improvement strategies for healthcare professionals who are involved in the revenue cycle.

As this book will be distributed nationally, some content is intended for general purposes only. For specific payer and state guidelines, we recommend contacting specific agencies and organizations for additional information. This manual includes sample documents, links to industry resources and knowledge checks to enhance your overall learning experience.

Throughout the book, we seek to provide options for incorporating quality payment programs, streamlined processes and tips for leveraging technology to optimize your revenue cycle building blocks. We also share guidance for uncovering missed financial opportunities within your practice's revenue cycle. We don't want you to just work the revenue cycle, we want you to master the revenue cycle! Happy reading.

Sincerely,
Taya and Kem

Chapter 1

Defining the Revenue Cycle Model (RCM)

The revenue cycle model (RCM) is the full process of billing and payment that takes place in healthcare facilities. Some view the RCM as the process from patient visit to claims payment, but the process is wider than that. RCM begins before the patient is seen and doesn't end until long after.

Once the basic components of RCM are in place and structurally sound, there are numerous ways to improve upon processes, decrease days in accounts receivable (A/R), and increase revenue. Like home construction, building a strong foundation is imperative. This book focuses on the basic building blocks of RCM.

What is RCM?

Depending on the context, RCM may stand for "revenue cycle model" or "revenue cycle management." The revenue cycle model, as stated above, refers to the full process of billing and payment that takes place in healthcare facilities. Revenue cycle management refers to the oversight and management of the revenue cycle. For the purposes of this book we will be addressing both.

At a high level, there are four main building blocks of the revenue cycle model:

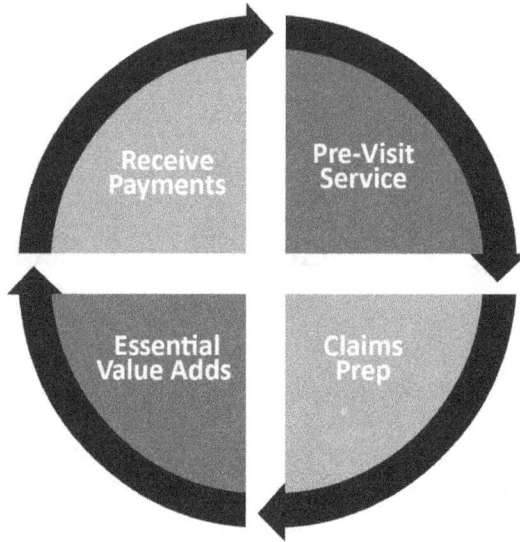

Figure 1.1

The cycle starts with pre-visit services, moves into claims preparation, then to receipt of payment and concludes with essential additional pieces that contribute to the success of the foundational blocks. In this book we will break out each of these sections into the full revenue cycle model shown below. In addition, we will include strategies, tips, and resources to help you succeed in RCM.

RCM Block by Block

This book will describe each step of the RCM in depth. Each chapter represents a building block that is critical to the foundation of your RCM.

Overlap

These blocks do not stand alone; there is quite a bit of overlap in each section. This overlap is by design, as each area of the RCM is interdependent. In some instances, we've highlighted the overlaps for you by indicating which chapter to refer to; in other instances, you can locate more information by navigating to the index.

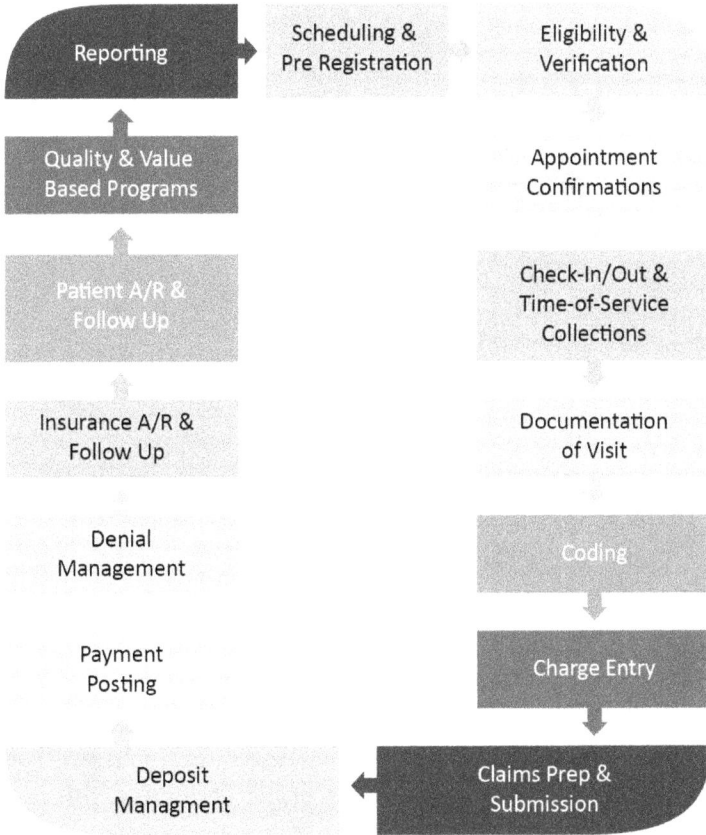

Figure 1.2 RCM Building Blocks

For example, patient eligibility and verification are foundational blocks of RCM. They are also critical components of pre-registration, check-in, prior authorizations, denial management, etc. Throughout the text there are many overlapping areas and intersecting touchpoints therefore we highly recommend using the index.

Scheduling & Pre-registration

This step is the first entry of the patient into the system. At each instance of patient contact, there is an opportunity to update demographic information. There are also opportunities to maximize provider's time by enhancing use of schedule templates and appointment scheduling.

Eligibility & Verification

In this step, practice staff verifies patient insurance information and coverage and determines benefits. Knowing patients benefits prior to service provides an opportunity for patient education and financial preparation.

Appointment Confirmations

Confirmations help improve show rates and capture last-minute information prior to the patient's face-to-face appointment.

Check-In/Check-Out & Time-of-Service

Patient check-in and check-out are the points where the patient enters and leaves the practice. During check-in, verify patient information is entered accurately into their electronic health record (EHR) and collect balances due, including copayments (copays). During check-out, schedule follow-up visits, verify alignment of services and charges, and provide a visit summary.

Documentation of Visit

Full documentation occurs after rendering services or during services when scribes are available. Documentation must include all services without gaps and should also include proper diagnoses information.

Coding

The coding of claims is a critical component of RCM and can directly cause significant penalties for the organization. Coding of procedures and diagnoses should always follow the most current edition of coding manuals issued for your specialty.

Charge Entry

Charges represent the fees for the services. Charge entry is the input of these fees into the practice management system to be submitted for payment.

Claims Preparation & Submission

The process of preparing a full claim and submitting an accurate claim, the first time, is essential.

Deposit Management

Deposit management processes ensure that all money is properly documented, reconciled, and deposited into the practice's accounts.

Payment Posting

The posting of payments and adjustments completes the claim cycle. Additionally, the payments posting process helps identify potential trends and changes in payments.

Denial Management

It is imperative to immediately review denials, appeal if appropriate, diagnose the root cause, and remediate to prevent future denials.

Insurance A/R & Follow-Up

After payment posting, there may be additional follow-up required to obtain full payment, such as submission to a secondary payer.

Patient A/R & Follow-Up

Patients may have a balance due in addition to the insurance payments. This could be the result of an outstanding deductible or a coinsurance amount due.

Reporting

Accurate reporting can lead to the identification of opportunities as well as problem areas. Reports are only as good as the data in the system and the parameters by which they're run.

Quality & Value-Based Program

As the industry shifts from fee-for-service to value-based payments, there is greater importance placed on quality program achievement. If your practice hasn't begun quality reporting yet, then you may be subject to unnecessary penalties.

RCM Challenges

Throughout the RCM process there will be challenges and pitfalls. In this book, we've included ways to turn stumbling blocks into opportunities to improve your revenue cycle. Stumbling blocks are not only financial, there will be operational-, technological-, and compliance-related challenges as well. The key is to plan-ahead for potential barriers and to optimize RCM strategy.

✐ Knowledge Check

Chapter 1: Defining the Revenue Cycle

Question #1:

The revenue cycle model can be divided into four main areas to manage. Name the four sections of the revenue cycle model:_____

_____

_____

Question #2:

The _____ process ensures that all money is properly documented, reconciled, and deposited into the practice's accounts.

Question #3:

The coding of claims is a critical RCM component, which is why you should always:_____

_____

_____

Answers

Q1: Pre-Visit Services, Claims Prep, Receive Payments, and Essential Add-ons.
Q2: Deposit management
Q3: Follow the most current edition of coding manuals issued for your specialty.

Chapter 2

Practice Preparation: Are You Planning to Fail?

It is said that if you fail to plan, you plan to fail. This is most definitely the case in RCM. Proper setup of providers, contracts, databases, and staffing are critical components of RCM success.

There are many challenges within the proper execution of RCM. Minimize the barriers to success by creating a solid foundation. A solid foundation includes proper credentialing, accurate system setup, and appropriate staffing. When the foundation is incomplete or set up incorrectly, gaps jeopardize the success and hinder the outcomes of best practices in the RCM.

Before diving into the other chapters, please review this preparatory section that provides strategies and considerations for new and established practices alike for reviewing foundational items that build a strong revenue model.

Practice Start Up

Business Plan and Checklist

Private practices that do not include the development of a business plan during the start-up phase of the organization might be missing a key structure that will guide their business. Many private practices have been, and continue to, operate as small businesses rather than as enterprises requiring formal structure. Bank funding or justification of capital purchases is the most common reason practices develop a business plan. Even then, the use of a business plan or new practice checklist is not always carried over to daily operations and strategic planning. A business plan and new practice checklist will include the original mission, vision, financial markers, checklist for tasks that require action and execution of goals for a practice.

A common line of thinking by physician owners is, "I'll hire people, treat patients, comply with regulations, bill insurance, get paid, pay bills, and be profitable." Obviously, this is an oversimplification, but not using a business plan, new practice checklist, or an implementation work plan will be to the potential detriment of the practice.

In time, the initial roadmap may change. The type of changes the practice experiences may conflict with the original plans. These changes may also be out of the control of the practice, such as, changing regulations, new programs, industry innovations, trends in population health management, care coordination, technology, and reimbursement requirements. If the original business plan or new practice checklist did not anticipate these changes, your practice may be unprepared or ill-equipped to manage a changing healthcare environment.

Whether you are working within a new or established practice, it's wise to take a step back and review your infrastructure. Working backwards to review previously established processes and map them to current and future needs may also yield results of previously unidentified missed steps or missed opportunities during practice set up.

There are times within the lifecycle of a practice that are great opportunities to circle back to the beginning and conduct a self-audit. Great opportunities to revisit an established practice's original business plan or start-up checklist or at least specific sections of a practice's original business plan may include:

Hiring: Providers, Leaders, Staff	Relocation	Acquisition or Merger
Change in revenue + or -	Outsourcing Services	Vendor Changes
Contract Negotiations	Adding Insurance participation	Change in EHR/PM Softwere
Incentive Program Participation	Audits	Identification of compliance issues

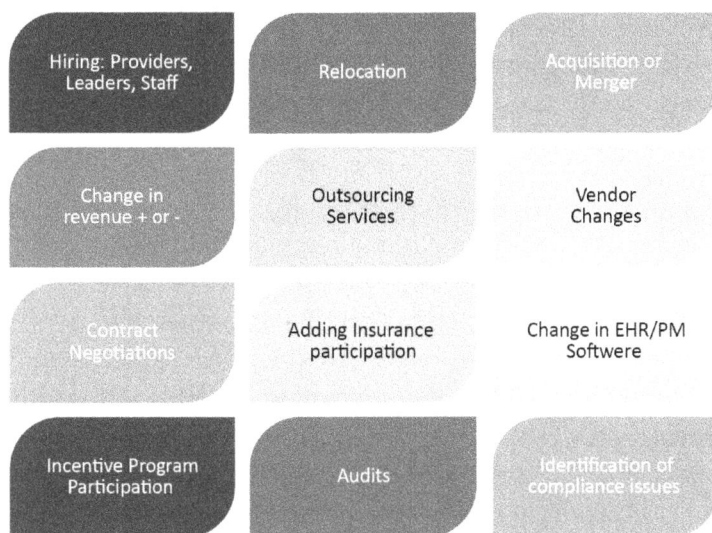

Figure 2.1   Opportunities to Revisit Business Plan or Practice Checklist

There are excellent resources to create a business plan. There are many online options, so exploring them to see if you can find one that works for your practice's needs and budget is probably worth the effort. In addition to resources for business plan development, MGMA has a helpful, "New Practice or Acquisition Start-up Checklist," that could be used for not only new practice start up or acquisition but also for self-auditing an existing practice.[1] You may also want to consider customizing your own practice assessment tool based on resources that might be available from your medical society, specialty medical organization, payroll management organization, HIT vendor, liability insurer, OIG, CMS or any other applicable organizations. Determine the areas within your practice that require review, identify and align your practice through membership, networking or other means to use external resources that are abreast of industry changes and provide best practice guidelines. In a telephone conversation, with a medical society, the following advice was given:

> As private medical practices strive to keep up with regulations, payment reform and industry best practices, alignment with organizations whose missions are to help them thrive will prove useful. The state medical societies are local medical practice

advocates. They provide support in the form of advocacy, training and education through CMEs, as well as practice support services. Consider taking a fresh look at your state medical society's resources and membership.

Gene Ransom, JD, CEO, MedChi, The Maryland State Medical Society

As you go through the process of reviewing and assessing your practice, consider sharing your plan or checklist with those staff members and providers responsible for executing these tasks. These key staff members can provide input into operationalizing steps that leaders may not have considered. Also, keep track of the areas that you are succeeding in as well as those that need improvement to develop a gap analysis.

A gap analysis can be used to improve workflows or add missed opportunities to your practice. It may also be used to assign previously unassigned tasks and include performance measures and accountability.

Insurance Credentialing

Raise your hand if you love credentialing! You know, waiting on hold for insurance companies, the pressure of your practice not getting paid for services due to non-participation. Don't all raise your hands at once! Whether you are with a new or established practice, it's always a good idea to revisit your participating payer records periodically to verify their records are accurate.

Without warning, payer's may update their records, which will impact your reimbursement. Take the following scenario, for example:

A Primary Care Physician (PCP) was enrolled with a large payer using the Family Medicine Taxonomy (207R00000X) as the primary taxonomy code. This physician was listed as a PCP for all her patients. Somehow, months after participation, the payer's records were modified, incorrectly switching the physician's second board certification of Emergency Medicine as the primary taxonomy code (207P00000X). Claims for preventive, primary care services were then denied.

Proactively confirming participation and enrollment may avoid incorrect processing. If provider demographic denials do occur, identify and address those credentialing issues quickly.

The process of insurance credentialing is different from the facility/hospital privileges credentialing process. Hospitals and facilities conduct a process of verifying a healthcare provider's credentials, background, history and qualifications prior to allowing them to have privileges to provide care. Insurance credentialing, from the healthcare provider's perspective, involves informing insurance companies that you're open for business, that you have clinical providers who are interested in treating their beneficiaries and receiving payment for healthcare services. Each insurance company has a verification or "credentialing" process that must be completed before they allow a healthcare provider to treat their members.

Primary Source Verification

Beginning in the 1990s, the (then) Joint Commission on Accreditation of Healthcare Organizations (JCAHO) required a primary source verification for licensed independent practitioners for acute care hospitals, which expanded to nurses and other healthcare providers, with the final expansion to ambulatory care settings by Joint Commission International (JCI).[2] Primary source verification is the process of verifying qualifications and credentials that have been presented by an individual directly with the source of that document or credential. This process of authenticating data, such as a medical degree, directly from the medical school or "primary source" is geared toward eliminating fraudulent representations of credentials and qualifications. Primary source verification may also be conducted through a designated equivalent source or an approved agent of the originating source who is able to provide identical information to the primary source.

Network Adequacy

The payer's credentialing processes include a review of their own network adequacy to ensure that they do not have too many or too few of a specific clinical specialty in each geographic region. There are times when a payer closes their network to specific specialties. Unique service offerings and a history of high-quality performance may help to grant an exception. Otherwise, request to have the organization added to the list of interested participants where possible.

Credentialing Process

A successful insurance credentialing process ends with participation and the ability to bill for services. This is accomplished with a contract or participation agreement with a fee schedule. To conclude the credentialing process be sure to agree upon the following items:

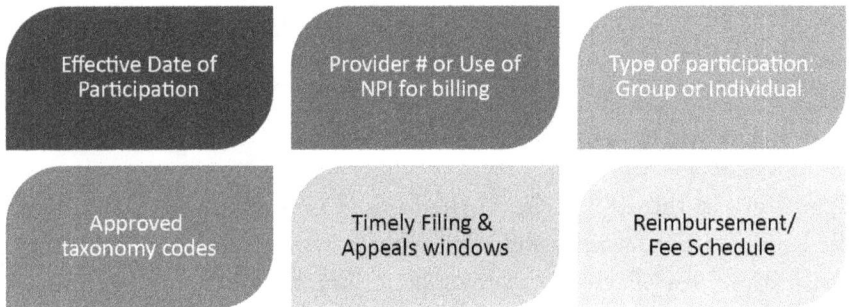

Effective Date of Participation	Provider # or Use of NPI for billing	Type of participation: Group or Individual
Approved taxonomy codes	Timely Filing & Appeals windows	Reimbursement/ Fee Schedule

Figure 2.2 Credentialing Process

As mentioned previously, there is a lack of uniformity in the insurance credentialing/enrollment process between payers. Some payers will have payer-specific forms and applications that must be completed for their health plans participation. It is vital that the payer-specific applications are completed by the practice in their entirety. If a payer imposes a deadline, do not delay completion and make sure to submit with proof of meeting the deadline (i.e., certified mail or return receipt). There are several payer-specific credentialing processes to be prepared for.

Table 2.1 Payer-Specific Credentialing Processes

Practice Assessment Form	Basic practice and provider information to include hours of operation, specialty-specific services, license information, ADA compliance.
Disclosure of Ownership	To avoid running afoul of Stark or anti-kickback statutes, payers must confirm practice ownership and identify any possible conflicts of interest.
Site Visit	It is common for certain Medicaid Managed Care Organizations (MCOs) to perform site visits that require a payer representative to visit the practice site to survey HIPAA compliance, exam rooms, laboratory, CLIA, ADA compliance, and other requirements.
Council for Affordable Quality Healthcare (CAQH)	Many payers regularly check the CAQH database to gather documents and confirm that licenses and liability insurance is valid.
Encrypted Messages	Some payers have strict security measures and will communicate via secured email. Be on the look-out in your junk e-mail folders for these payer communications to avoid missing vital messages.
DocuSign	To expedite the contracting process, some payers may opt for electronic signatures on contracts. DocuSign® is one vendor that is used for this purpose. Regularly check junk e-mail folders for these communications.
Original Signatures	There are instances in which payers require an original signature on applications and contracts. Consider having blue ink used for these purposes. When mailing documents to payers, use some type of document tracker such as FedEx® or certified return receipt.
Notarized Contracts	Anticipate that there are payers that require notarized contracts. Ensure that you follow their guidelines for these requests.

Keep copies of every document, application, and communication with an insurance company during the credentialing process and date the transmittal whether through mail or electronic. When performing online credentialing, consider grabbing a print screen of your application and saving it in your files.

New practices or new physicians will need to consider having certain business infrastructure in place prior to initiating the credentialing process. Some payers may request a letter of intent to participate on the practice's letterhead. Normally practice stationery isn't finalized until a logo and website have been created. Consider using a makeshift header as a temporary letterhead for the purpose of a letter of intent.

The practice must have proof of liability coverage, a phone, fax, tax identification number (TIN), organizational National Provider Identifier (NPI) number, practice location, and pay-to address to initiate the credentialing process. Using a temporary phone and fax number is permissible, however, keep in mind that going in this direction will disrupt the practice's communication with the payer in the future as it takes time to update payer's records with new practice contact information.

Insurance Linking

If the providers you are performing insurance credentialing for have been (1) actively treating patients, (2) participating with insurances within the state that you are seeking to credential them for the TIN of your practice, or, (3) have recently completed the re-credentialing process for the respective payer; some payers will bypass the full credentialing process and use a linking process. The linking process usually occurs while the provider is still an active participating provider within the health plan. In some instances, the linking process is completed faster than the initial credentialing process.

Insurance Linking Scenario

Doctor is resigning from his group practice employment to start his own medical practice under his new TIN. He has been participating with all the major local insurance plans for years under his employer's TIN and has recently been re-credentialed with several payers under his employer's TIN. His current employer has not yet terminated his payer participation under their group TIN and payer contracts.

Doctor's new practice staff informs the major local insurance plans that he wishes to participate under a new TIN. The insurance companies are informed that the physician has a new practice location, pay-to address and organizational NPI. If applicable, the insurance companies will confirm their records and link the physician to the new organization. The linking process may not follow the standard initial credentialing process, however, the physician should be disassociated with the former TIN at an agreed upon date and participating with a new contract under the new TIN.

Insurance Credentialing Timeline

In the credentialing process, timing is everything. When you are preparing to begin insurance credentialing, you should also consider timing and non-uniformity. It will take time to credential or panel a provider with a payer. Each payer has their own process for insurance credentialing, so there is a lack of uniformity that requires a thorough understanding of each payer's credentialing requirements and timelines. Payers will not guarantee a timeline; however, most payers tell practices to expect a 120-day (4 month) credentialing timeline.

Although healthcare providers it is tempting, resist the urge to begin treating patients before the credentialing and contracting processes are completed. During the phase of requesting to participate, request an effective date that aligns with the date you would like the physician to begin treating patients. Some payers may not honor or approve retroactive effective dates, so it's best to be aware of these rules prior to providing care.

As you consider the appropriate credentialing timeline for your practice, keep in mind external entities that will need to use your enrollment information to make sure you are paid. Two entities that will rely on your enrollment information and that should be factored into your credentialing timeline are your Clearinghouse and Practice Management software.

Once the insurance credentialing process is completed, your clearinghouse and practice management (PM) software will need to prepare their systems to accept and manage claim scrubbing, claim edits, claim submission, posting of Electronic Remittance Advice (ERA), and Electronic Funds Transfers (EFT). In many instances, the clearinghouse has a bi-directional interface with the PM software, or the PM software has their own built-in clearinghouse.

The time needed for these entities to perform their own payer verification and enrollment processes should be factored into your overall credentialing timeframe. Expect a four- to six-week timeframe. However, this varies, so check with your clearinghouse and PM software vendor to find out their required timeline for their enrollment processes. Incorporate all these factors when setting an appropriate practice go-live or date to begin treatment: it should be timed for after credentialing, payer contracting, and software or clearinghouse enrollment are completed.

In the event the practice begins treating patients prior to software or clearinghouse enrollment is completed, there is a likelihood that payments and remittance advice may not be sent to the practice electronically. If a third party is responsible for payment posting and denial management, processes will need to be in place for the practice to securely send paper remittance advice and payment information to the third party for posting claims correction, when applicable, and payment reconciliation.

Again, each payer has their own unique credentialing process and timeline. It is recommended that you understand the credentialing and contracting guidelines for each payer before you begin the process. Consider obtaining the below information from the payer before getting started:

- Direct contact information (phone, fax, email, website) for the credentialing or provider enrollment department or representative
- Average timeline for completion of the credentialing and contracting processes
- Direct contact person or department for the contracting process (phone, fax, email, website)
- Manner in which the practice may request participation (i.e., CAQH, payer's website, letter on practice letterhead)

As you are factoring timelines from credentialing to participation, the steps listed below provide a basic overview of a typical credentialing process.

Preparation

The credentialing process is continuous and even if your practice uses a system like CAQH, you should retain provider demographic information in a provider file for permanent reference. Unfortunately, not all providers will be a lifer at your organization, which means you may one day lose access to their CAQH profile. A Provider Credentialing Questionnaire is a useful tool for collecting and keeping critical demographic data from your providers. A template is provided as Appendix B, and it can aid you in capturing key pieces of information that will be needed for the credentialing process.

Each state and insurance company will have their own requirements and documents necessary for credentialing. This questionnaire may be used to assist in gathering necessary information prior to starting the credentialing process. It may take time to obtain required documentation, so using this questionnaire as an inventory of what is needed and what is on file will put you in good standing to start the insurance credentialing process. Please see the back of the book for a sample Provider Credentialing Questionnaire.

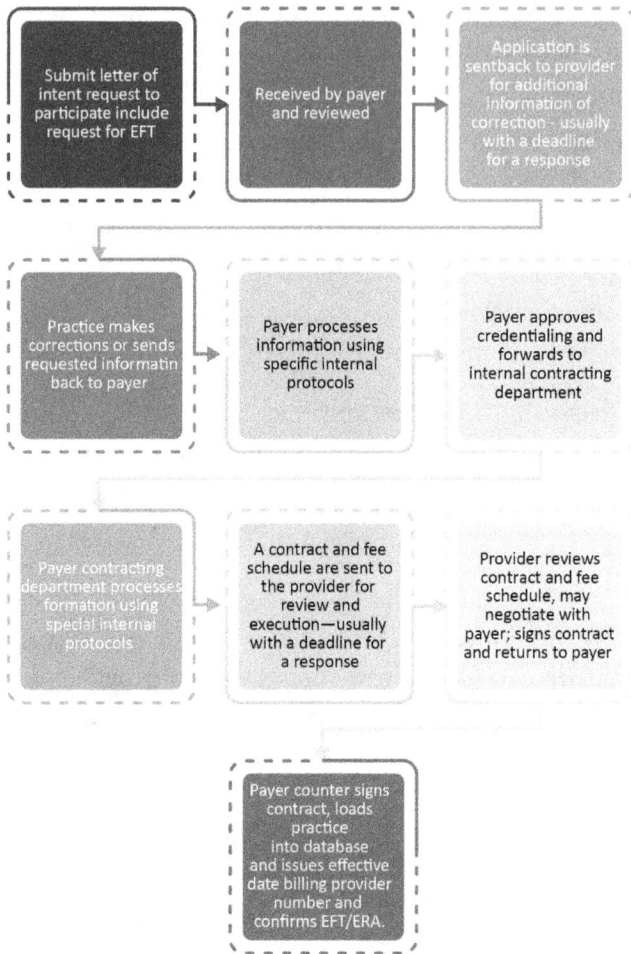

Figure 2.3   Typical Credentialing Process

Credentialing Matrix

During the credentialing process, documentation of conversations, reference numbers, payer contact information, the status of credentialing, action items, and communications should occur.

Documentation should include the name of the individuals you are speaking with, including their titles.

Target Payer List	Outline of all payers that will be included in credentialing
Timeline	Amount of time it generally may take to credential vs initial treatment date
Summary	Description of credentialing status for all payers
Practice & Provider Info	Pertinent info needed about the practice and providers: Tax ID#, NPI#s, Taxonomy's, License info, practice and pay to address Phone, fax, email, names of key payer representatives and departments
Payer Contact Info	Phone, fax, email, names of key payer representative and departments
Payer Communications	Documentation of all communications with payer to include names, dates, reference/case
Payer Contracts	Outline of all contracts on file, effective and expiration dates, key terms and conditions, fee schedules
Time Filing	Timeframe for practice to submit claims to payer from the date of service

Figure 2.4   Credentialing Matrix Information Tracking

The representative should be able to provide you with a reference or case number and should be able to confirm whether your application is complete. If the application is not complete the representative may be able to provide a description of specific items needed for completion along with deadlines where applicable. The next steps for the application and the timeline they anticipate for the application to be completed are key items to confirm. Additionally, the representative may be able to confirm if they will honor your requested effective date.

It is fundamental to have this information accessible to necessary members within the practice and for the person responsible for credentialing. If your practice does not use a credentialing software, then consider keeping all pertinent information in one document. This tool will aid in successfully documenting and tracking the insurance credentialing progress.

The information being stored is confidential and proprietary, so implementing security measures such as encryption, password protection, and user controls for such a document are essential. Only individuals who are authorized to see and use this information need access, limiting access only to these individuals will help avoid a data breach. When documenting conversations with insurance companies, the devil is in the details, so be as detailed as possible in your documentation, as it may be required to justify your position throughout the process.

A central location to track the entire credentialing process allows for accountability for practice and payer task completion, proof of actions completed, and talking points when checking the status of completion. Your state's Insurance Commissioner may have standards and requirements for payers to complete the insurance credentialing process. If so, including those guidelines in your matrix will help to better inform your staff.

Navigating Credentialing Databases

There are several go-to databases for provider credentialing. The most frequently used include:

- EIDM
  - CMS' Enterprise Identity Management system
- I&A
  - CMS' Identity & Access Management system[3]

- PECOS
  - Medicare's Provider Enrollment, Chain, and Ownership System
- NPPES
  - The CMS National Plan and Provider Enumeration System[4]
- CAQH
  - Council for Affordable Quality Healthcare

Each of these databases provides its own benefit and many require unique logins, though there has been some consolidation of logins in the last few years.

EIDM and I&A

The Centers for Medicare & Medicaid Services (CMS) Identity & Access Management System (I&A) is where providers should manage their identity and any authorized or delegated officials who may process documents or otherwise work within CMS systems on the provider's behalf[5]. This information updates the provider's CMS' Enterprise Identity Management (EIDM) system profile, which acts as a single-sign-on point of access to PECOS, NPPES, and the EHR Incentive portal. CMS takes security seriously. Be aware that authorized and delegated officials (individuals who are not the provider of care) will need to provide personal demographic information to access this database. This may include a social security number and date of birth. There may also be the requirement of agreeing to an identity verification process.

In order to create an EIDM account, the provider will need their I&A information, basic demographic information, NPI, and PTAN. The PTAN is the provider's unique identifier as a Medicare participant and stands for Provider Transaction Access Number.[6] The PTAN is issued to providers by Medicare Administrative Contractors (MACs) upon enrollment.

> If you have questions on setting up an EIDM, visit: https://portal.cms.gov/wps/portal/unauthportal/help/

PECOS

Medicare's provider enrollment is performed through their Provider Enrollment, Chain, and Ownership System, generally referred to as PECOS. Put simply, PECOS is the electronic means for updating provider enrollment information. This is where providers document locations, services, supervised or supervising providers, license information, and more. This where Medicare will reference provider credentialing information. To learn more about PECOS or create an account, navigate to: https://pecos.cms.hhs.gov/pecos/login.do#headingLvl.

NPPES

The National Plan & Provider Enumeration System (NPPES) assigns unique 10-digit numbers to providers and health plans for identification purposes. Like PECOS, you can log into NPPES with your EIDM account. It is very important that the taxonomy code you document here is accurate to the services you provide. The NPPES registry is a point of reference for many payer databases and inaccuracies here can lead to payment issues. Upon completion, the provider will be issued a National Provider Identifier (NPI).[7] This identifier will be used on all credentialing documents as well as all claims. Document this number as soon as it has been confirmed and double-check the accuracy of this number at any point of entry.

An NPI is also required for practices. This number is referred to as a Type 2 Organizational NPI. This identifier is also obtained through the NPPES. For more information on the NPI registry and the NPPES, navigate to https://nppes.cms.hhs.gov/webhelp/nppeshelp/NPPES%20FAQS.html.

CAQH

The Council for Affordable Quality Healthcare (CAQH) created a database they dubbed the Universal Provider Data source (UPD).[8]

CAQH's UPD is one of the most useful resources for those responsible for provider credentialing. When setting up the provider's profile in the UPD, pay close attention to data entered and double-check all fields. This is a comprehensive provider profile where you will input demographics, education, licenses, provider identifiers, payer enrollment IDs, locations, hours, contact numbers, specialty information, malpractice coverage, and other key credentialing information.

Upon completion, the system will require upload of key documents and attestation of data entered. Once this has been completed, the practice can grant access to participating payers. This is an immeasurable time-savings for staff, as payers will use this resource to re-credential providers instead of sending separate forms for completion. To get started with CAQH, navigate to: https://proview.caqh.org/.

Notably, Medicare revalidations must still be performed directly through PECOS[9]. For more information on Medicare Revalidations, navigate to https://www.cms.gov/Medicare/Provider-Enrollment-and-Certification/MedicareProviderSupEnroll/Downloads/Reval_Cycle2_FAQs.pdf.

COMPUTER Callout: Credentialing is a great example of a situation which can be substantially optimized through technology. Credentialing staff and specialists should be educated in the processes for updating CAQH profiles as well as other payer portal profiles. For example, though Medicare revalidations must be performed through the PECOS portal, the development of this electronic process provides a much quicker process than Medicare's paper revalidation form packet which can be quite lengthy to complete.[10]

Taxonomy

The importance of proper use and selection of taxonomy codes cannot be understated. CMS describes taxonomy codes as:

> The Healthcare Provider Taxonomy Code Set is a hierarchical code set that consists of codes, descriptions, and definitions. Healthcare Provider Taxonomy Codes are designed to categorize the type, classification, and/or specialization of health care providers. The Code Set consists of two sections: Individuals and Groups of Individuals, and Non-Individuals.[11]

As if we didn't need more codes to contend with, taxonomy codes are alphanumeric with ten characters. Double-check the use of taxonomy codes to avoid missing characters. HIPAA 5010 compliance requires the use of taxonomy codes as well as the use of NPIs. The many code sets being used in healthcare allow us to securely transmit, receive, and store protected health information (PHI).

There are two categories of taxonomy codes: "individuals" and "non-individuals." Either code category may include single specialty or multi-specialty providers. Confirm the applicable taxonomy category for your provider or practice.

Taxonomy Categories

Individuals 17 subcategories including but not limited to	Non-Individuals 11 subcategories including but not limited to
Physicians	Hospitals
Dental Providers	Laboratories
Dietary & Nutrition Service Providers	MCs
Nursing Service Providers	Nursing & Custodial Care Facilities
Physician Assistants	Transportation Services

During the NPI set up on the NPPES database, selection of taxonomy codes is required. We've learned that there are two types of NPIs: *Individual* and *Organization*. A taxonomy code is tagged to the respective NPI for additional classification. The taxonomy code provides a descriptor of the specialization and type of healthcare provider or entity tied to the NPI being used. Taxonomy codes are self-selected, meaning the provider or their representative selects their own taxonomy codes. To provide a level of accuracy, consider having the provider involved in the process of selecting taxonomy codes. It is also important to note that a provider may select more than one taxonomy; just be sure to sequence the primary taxonomy code first as the main specialty. Although professional organizations and credentialing boards provide the definitions for taxonomy codes, there is no requirement the provider be certified in the respective specialty.

The National Uniform Claim Committee (NUCC) updates the taxonomy codes twice a year: April 1 and October 1.[12] With the bi-annual updates to these codes, there is the possibility that the taxonomy codes you selected will become out of date. Code accuracy will impact provider specialty designation, which may in turn impact claims payments. For this reason, you will want to check taxonomy codes regularly. There are online resources available for searching taxonomy codes. The Code Set is available from the Washington Publishing Company (WPS). This URL links to a taxonomy look up: http://www.wpc-edi.com/reference/codelists/healthcare/health-care-provider-taxonomy-code-set/.

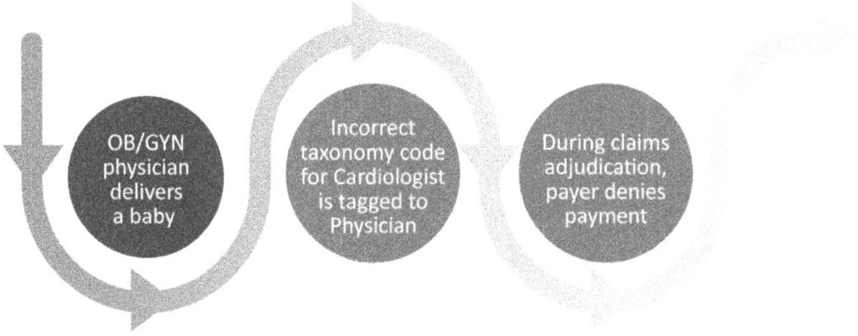

Figure 2.6 Taxonomy Claims Processing Scenario

Payers are using taxonomy codes for a host of purposes. They are determining network adequacy, appropriateness of care and claims adjudication.

Correct use of taxonomy codes assists with accurate and timely claims processing. Below is an example of how a taxonomy code appears on a claim form.[13]

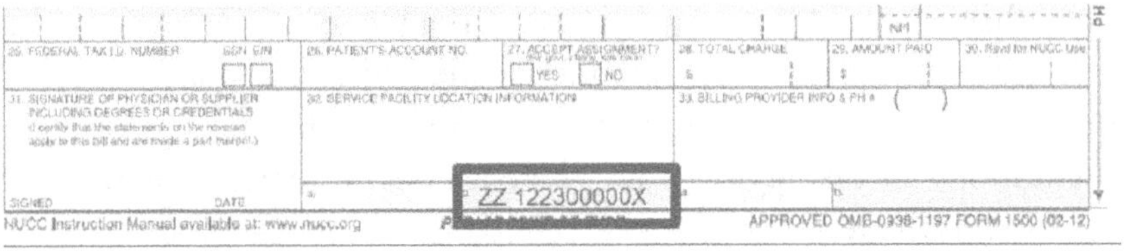

Figure 2.7   Example taxonomy code on a claim form

Impact of EHR on RCM

Who remembers the "good old days" of paper charts? You know, the carbon copy message pads? Pulling charts for the day's appointments? Filing, yes filing, all those charts and, heaven forbid, a misfiled chart resulted in someone created a new chart for an existing patient. Printing a boatload of superbills and highlighting key information? Even better, printing Health Care Finance Administration (HCFA) claim forms and having bales of mail to process? Fun times, right? Not so much. Since those paper charts have been replaced with electronic health records, misfiling an entire chart is pretty much eliminated. The message pad has been replaced with secure internal messaging. Superbills are all but obsolete, and it is the new norm for claims to be submitted electronically.

Even those who aren't EHR cheerleaders can agree that innovation is necessary. Healthcare sees more change in any six-month period than many industries see in years. According to the ONC,

Our world has been radically transformed by digital technology – smart phones, tablets, and web-enabled devices have transformed our daily lives and the way we communicate. Medicine is an information-rich enterprise. A greater and more seamless flow of information within a digital health care infrastructure, created by electronic health records (EHRs), encompasses and leverages digital progress and can transform the way care is delivered and compensated.[14]

As practices are transitioning from paper to EHR and PM software, RCM processes are changing as well. Find out if your EHR/PM software has a mobile app for staff as well as patients.

Below is an example of how EHR / PM software has impacted RCM:

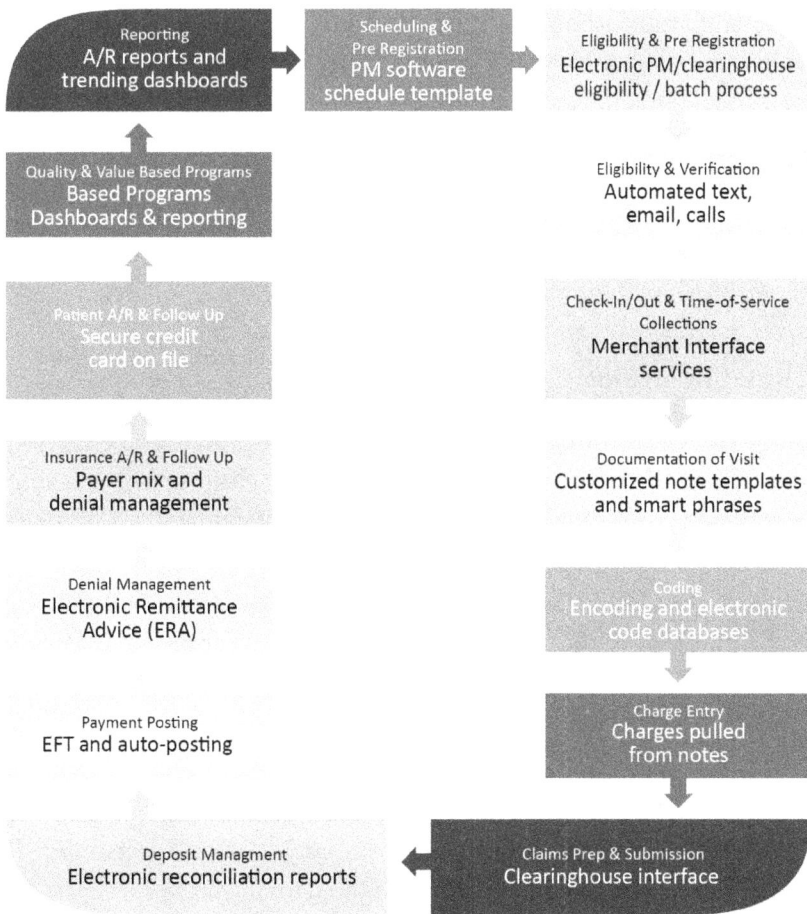

Figure 2.8   EHR and PM software impact on RCM

Implementing an EHR/PM System

Time and resources must be devoted to a successful EHR and PM software implementation. The lack of proper set up will have negative impacts on the user experience, functionality of the software, and bottlenecks in the overall RCM. As described in the above graphic, your software has an impact on every building block of the RCM. Let's discuss factors necessary for a successful software implementation.

Project Manager and Champions

Someone must steer the ship. Select someone within your practice to oversee and troubleshoot the entire EHR/PM software implementation. This individual should have higher-level authority to make decisions on behalf of the practice, as well as have an overall knowledge of all areas of the practice. They will also be coordinating activities on behalf of the practice with the software company's implementation specialist. The practice will need team members to support the project manager. These champions would most likely be physicians or other providers who also have decision-making authority.

Practice Information

During an EHR implementation, practice information needs to be entered into the software accurately. Each customized section of the software uses practice information for varying and sometimes overlapping purposes. For example, correctly entering practice's pay to address into the software will ensure that insurance payments from electronic claims submissions are sent to the correct location. Accurately entering provider Drug Enforcement Administration (DEA) numbers into the software will facilitate electronic prescribing capabilities through the software interface.

Bad data in is bad data out, so be sure that practice information being entered or given to your software company is 100% accurate. This information includes the practice's legal name, all NPIs, Controlled Dangerous Substance (CDS) and state licenses, phone, fax, website, email, and other public facing information. The software company should provide a list of required practice data for entry. Determine whether you prefer to enter your practice data directly into the software yourself, or to have the software company enter it for you. Either way, validate all practice information and conduct testing using practice information prior to going live.

As you are providing your software vendor with your practice information, it's also a good idea to obtain their resource list assigned to your practice or general departments that your practice may need to reach. Maintaining a software resource list should include contacts that will guide practice employees who have questions to the appropriate software representative. A resource list does not have to be complex; it may simply include the name, title, role in implementation, email, and phone numbers for everyone from the practice and software vendor who will be actively participating in the software implementation.

The individuals championing the software implementation on behalf of the practice should maintain these reference documents for future use. There might be turnover of software employees so be sure to make updates to contact lists as needed.

Within the practice, it's important to have internal access controls by monitoring practice user software access and permissions. This may be done by creating a list of users which includes the name, title, role in the practice, software access needs and levels, department, and training requirements of all staff members who will need software access.

Other information that will be helpful prior to, during and after software implementation is a software quick-reference guide. This guide will provide an overview of software functionality, software features that the practice is using, pricing and practice hardware needs.

Master Project Plan

How will you know if you're meeting deadlines for software implementation? How would you keep track of software implementation tasks in addition to your other daily practice responsibilities? The answer is the use of a master project plan. Ask your vendor if they have a template that you can use. If not, create one yourself. The purpose of a master project plan is for you (the practice champion) to keep track of the tasks, deliverables, outcomes, and overall status of your EHR/PM software implementation and go-live. Failure to track outcomes may delay your anticipated go-live date or delay enabling or optimizing key software features. This will result in a poor end user experience. Having a master project plan is also helpful after go-live in the event issues arise; you can look-back at the plan to see where something may have fallen through the cracks. It's also helpful to have it available for new employees who are taking over as an EHR/PM software super user so they can track implementation steps and identify areas that need to be improved.

The plan should be available for review and even updating by necessary stakeholders. Include important dates, deadlines, task assignments and responsible parties, priority levels of tasks, contingencies, and status of tasks. This information should be reviewed and updated regularly to anticipate problems and find solutions to staying on target. Consider color coding responsibilities by practice and by software vendor.

MGMA has excellent guides for resources and project planning EHR implementations, additionally most EHR vendors also provide project planning tools after contract signature.

Portal Interfaces

Most EHR/PM software does not stand alone. They are linked to other platforms to provide interoperability for their clients. For example, EHR/PM software's typically do not have their own ability to connect with pharmacies electronically. As healthcare providers have a strong need to manage medications within the EHR, the software agrees to interface with a platform that has these unique capabilities. The EHR/PM software will interface with an ePrescribing platform such as SureScripts for secure ePrescribing, medication management and formulary information.

There are many other interfaces or connections that the EHR/PM software may develop based on their own limitations and based on practice needs. Determine your software's capabilities compared to your practice's workflows to identify your required interfaces and present them to your vendor. These interface needs may include laboratories for orders in and orders out, physician to physician (P2P) communications, immunization registry, health information exchange (HIE), radiology, telecommunications, clinical equipment, and clearinghouse. Some interfaces are transaction volume driven, so be sure to investigate costs.

If your PM software is separate from your EHR, that would be a priority interface. To keep all information flowing between both your EHR and PM systems, request a bi-directional interface. This eliminates the need of entering patient information twice; once in the EHR and then again in the PM software. When selecting an EHR/PM software determine whether you require an open application programming interface (API). This allows greater flexibility with interfacing with other software. Many EHR/PM software do not permit an API but rather have preferred add-on software platforms that they will permit for interfacing. Request a list of these platforms to compare with internal practice needs. Keep a list of all required technology portal interfaces, methods of connection to the EHR, both internal and external. This is helpful in the event an interface stops working so you can follow up and troubleshoot.

Hardware Specifications and Inventory

When using EHR/PM software there will be specific hardware needs. There might be certain devices that may not be compatible with your software. Performing a hardware inventory prior to purchase will determine future hardware needs. Also keep track of current and future hardware purchases, documenting operating system requirements from the EHR/PM software company. Hardware requirements, such as scanners and copiers that can work efficiently with the software, should be assessed for all functional areas of the organization.

During your assessment and review, consider hardware that needs to be replaced or purchased to optimize practice workflow. For example, would you like laptops to be used in exam rooms to assist nursing staff with documenting patient vital signs and providers with documenting encounter visit notes while providing care? If so, determine whether you have the correct number of available laptops for practice users. Talk to your information technology (IT) vendor about required device cabling, networking devices, and hardware requirements to meet HIPAA security requirements. Based on staff roles, the hardware necessary to optimize workflows may vary, including mobile workstations, insurance and ID card scanners, credit card readers, cameras for taking patient pictures and adding to profiles, and mobile check-in devices for self-registration. Most EHRs are capable of faxing, but that may not eliminate the need for a free-standing fax machine. Conducting an inventory of needs based on your optimal practice workflow will allow you to have necessary hardware devices to optimize the use of your EHR/PM software.

Templates and forms

Practice forms such as intake, consent, authorizations, financial policy, medical history, registration, and notice of privacy practices can be integrated into EHRs. Providers will have individual needs for customized progress note templates based on diagnosis, specialty, and service type. Some specialty associations will provide template tips. The goal for templates is to include fields necessary for capturing complete and accurate medical record documentation. Sometimes secondary modules are available to add-on features like transcription. Since providers are primary users of the templates and forms, including them in the process provides a platform to gain their input as to generic and customizable software options. The use of preventive medicine questionnaires should also be available and customizable. Some software vendors have pre-developed industry standard templates such as the Patient Health Questionnaire-9 (PHQ-9) depression screening, Annual Wellness Visit (AWV), Chronic Care Management (CCM), Medical Orders for Life Sustaining Treatment form (MOLST), Advance Directives, and Health Risk Assessment (HRA). Again, confirm whether your software has public forms already established.

Billing and Collections

Evaluate the software's capability for claim submission and related costs. Sometimes EHR and PM software packages are bundled by the vendor and include billings/collections service. In these circumstances, the vendor then agrees to take over the management of billing and collections on behalf of the practice. Essentially, this option would replace the need for certain internal billing and collections staff. It is however; recommended to have practice personnel oversee the operations of any form of outsourced billing and collections.

Outsourcing billing and collections to your software vendor will include a fee, which is typically a percentage of the practice's financial collections. Software vendor fees typically range from 3% to 13%.[15] The rate payable by the practice to the software vendor depends on factors such as volume, specialty, payer mix and complexity. This fee may or may not include software user licenses and other ancillary fees.

In addition to billing and collections services, practices will encounter patients who have been given notice of outstanding bills and practice collections efforts have been exhausted. These cases may require turning over patient accounts to a bad debt agency. In the event you decide to use a bad debt collections agency, consider whether an interface or access to the agencies software will be required to be able to securely transmit patient demographics, insurance and identification cards, financial liability attestations, and other related information to your agency for follow up. This is also a good time to determine user access levels and permissions, especially when it comes to permission to write off or adjust balances.

The configuration of a PM system is fundamental to the success of the organization. Taking the time to set the software up correctly means entering accurate data for providers and the practice. It also means accurate mapping of code set and adjustment codes. The implementation of a PM system usually takes many steps, including setup of patient statement letters, insurance groups and more, some of this information ties in directly to the EHR. The project manager for the implementation or the software vendor should have a list of necessary and recommended action steps for setup.

Payer Enrollment Process

Your PM software may have their own built in clearinghouse; if not, then it may interface with a clearinghouse. You will want to have a bi-directional interface between your PM software and clearinghouse. Either way, in order to initiate the billing process, your clearinghouse will need to enroll your practice through their software using your credentialing and payer enrollment information. This enrollment process will require the practice to provide the PM software or clearinghouse with payer welcome letters. If welcome letters are not available, check with your clearinghouse or PM software vendor for a complete list of their enrollment requirements.

The enrollment process will allow the software company to initiate an Electronic Data Interchange (EDI) with each payer for claim submission, ERAs, and EFTs. This data will populate business reports in the PM software. During the credentialing process, it will be necessary to request ERA and EFT and include your clearinghouse in these discussions for potential coordination. Included in the clearinghouse set up is the eligibility (270/271) set up which allows your staff to verify patient insurance eligibility directly in the PM software.[16]

Dashboard Utilization for Performance Measures

In the event your practice is participating in quality programs or documenting preventive medicine services, you'll want to keep track of performance measures for program reporting. This can be easily tracked through canned system reports or dashboards which meet program standards and capture necessary tracking information. These dashboards should also give the user the ability to take corrective actions as needed. The overall goal of dashboards is to allow the practice to visualize program performance and areas for improvement. Software vendors often offer training to learn how to properly populate these dashboards from within the system.

Reporting

To manage the financial health of a medical practice, it's critical to have access to actionable data. Development of key financial reports is essential to this process. Countless decisions will be made based upon this information, from service expansion, to staffing models, to compensation, as well as ensuring compliance. Financial information is also important to external business partners, including financial institutions, lenders, and government agencies. In Chapter 15, we discuss reporting in further detail. Software vendors are the best resource for understanding customization capabilities. For example, your software may have canned reports as well as custom reports. Some software vendors request the practice to complete a form outlining reporting needs in either case, clearly communicate your needs and request specific training for report use.

Patient Engagement

Communication with patients is key in population health, care plan compliance, and chronic illness management, which all serve to improve care quality and lower care costs. EHRs can allow us to provide patient education and accept online payments. The use of an EHR allows for secure and innovative patient engagement through awareness and outreach campaigns. Seasonal health campaigns such as flu clinics or disease reminders for chronic illnesses can be accomplished in a secure environment via a patient portal, encrypted messages, and practice websites. The practice may also monitor and improve the patient experience through surveys such as the Consumer Assessment of Healthcare Providers & Systems° (CAHPS). Patient experience is included in quality programs, so optimize your software's patient engagement features to meet these goals. While building out your patient portal, there are settings that will need to be configured, such as intake and consent forms, appointment scheduling, email messages, security, and access. Configuring settings based on your practice workflows and training staff to educate patients on use takes time but pays off.

Test Environment

Some vendors offer EHR/PM software test environments to practice using all features prior to going live on the software. The test environment will allow you to use features without permanently making changes. This is helpful to find gaps and make mistakes prior to using the software in a real environment. Several functions to run in a test environment would be registering a patient, entering a charge, documenting a visit, documenting vitals, creating a claim, and scheduling an appointment. Navigating through a test environment and performing mock trials of processes is an excellent learning opportunity.

Training and Education

Many EHR/PM software companies have created virtual environments for software training. These environments include live web-based training, recorded training, You-Tube channels, and training manuals. Sometimes, the best option for training your workforce is a hybrid of available learning methods and platforms. Some key moments to offer training include before going live with a software, hiring of new staff and providers, software upgrades, or new software features. It doesn't hurt to periodically retrain staff on software features that are being underutilized or being used incorrectly. For an additional fee, most software companies will provide onsite training. Prior to initiating software training, create a software training checklist based on user roles with your software company to avoid missing any key software training. Most practices will have a super user who has been trained on all features of the software implementation to be the go-to person internally. Conducting knowledge checks for all users can ensure that they comprehend and can apply the training provided.

Workflow Mapping

Mapping practice workflows to EHR/PM software capabilities is a key component of a successful implementation. Failure to map workflows may lead to end user frustration if they cannot conduct daily operations because necessary functions were not built out in the software in advance. Current workflows should be identified and documented for reference. Document the new process that will be integrated into the EHR/PM software, determine if a process improvement plan (PIP) is required, and map out the new PIP.

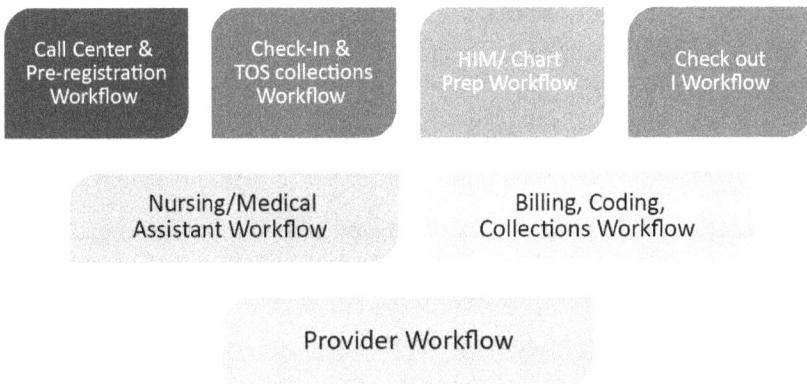

Call Center & Pre-registration Workflow	Check-In & TOS collections Workflow	HIM/ Chart Prep Workflow	Check out I Workflow
	Nursing/Medical Assistant Workflow	Billing, Coding, Collections Workflow	
	Provider Workflow		

Figure 2.9   Workflows to Consider for Improvement

Security

With any internet-based platform, there are security risks. As we continuously strive to build relationships and trust with our patients, we want to provide a transparent security environment to put the public at ease. Security risk assessments (SRA) must be completed annually for covered entities. Practices are obligated to keep patients informed about how their protected health information (PHI) is being managed, stored and shared. The notice of privacy practices (NPP) is a required posting. Due to the sensitive nature of the information being stored, transmitted, and received within the EHR/PM software, we must take precautions to safeguard the confidentiality of this information. Role-based access, encryption, network security, monitoring access, and constant workforce education are good lines of defense. Patient Security Access Codes

(PSAC) should be developed and used to protect the privacy of specific patient's names and PHI. Some patient names will be required to be confidential, such as employees who are patients, patients who request name confidentiality, and public figures. Other patients may prefer that their real name not be distributed to others, such as family members.

User access controls are a primary factor for EHR/PM software security. User access can be defined and restricted based on function. Roles and access require review in the software and map to internal staffing requirements. Access should fit the role, no more and no less. Upon employment termination, access should also be terminated. Access to PHI should be defined in compliance with HIPAA requirements.

Data Migration

The migration of PHI and data from one software to another is a step that automatically populates your new EHR/PM software with prior records and information. The new system vendor should provide a list of the file formats acceptable by the distributing and receiving software companies. Many will use a CSV file. There are limitations to what type of data can be migrated from one software to another. Important data files for migration include patient demographics and corresponding insurance information, as well as any related images such as insurance cards and picture IDs. You'll also want to migrate patient records and related images such as external reports. Depending on your ability to access old A/R, you may want to start fresh in your new PM software; however, if possible, it's a good idea to determine the capability of exporting old A/R to include insurance and patient balances and account notes into the new software. Working down legacy A/R might be best accomplished in your old system. There should be a cut-off date that differentiates new and old A/R for tracking.

Fee Schedules

Many software companies will provide the practice with a template to populate a Charge Description Master (CDM) that will list all the

CPT and HCPCS codes used by a practice, along with the practice's charge amount for each service. In addition to your charge amount, which is typically different from the allowed amounts that each payer will reimburse, you'll also want to consider uploading the allowable amounts from your payer fee schedules into your PM software. Doing so allows for accurate payment posting. If an incoming insurance payment is posted below or above the payer's allowed amount, an alert will be provided from the software making the user aware that there is a problem. If an alert is generated, action should be taken to address the variance. Unfortunately, some staff may ignore these alerts, so it is helpful to have a process for monitoring actions taken on alerts payment posting errors.

There is never a time limit to reviewing your EHR/PM software features and capabilities and matching them to your practice's current needs. Doing so will allow you to optimize the use of the software to reduce administrative burdens and improve user experience.

Staffing for Success

Education

Staffing for success begins with ensuring staff have the right knowledge, skill set, and behaviors to accomplish the goals of your practice. This doesn't necessarily mean that everyone has a master's degree in health care administration. Sometimes the employees are homegrown, meaning they received on the job training instead of formal training. In many circumstances, practices prefer homegrown staff, promoting the front desk receptionist up the staffing hierarchy to management. Opportunity for professional advancement is significant, as is the opportunity to work with long-term staff that you trust. However, this approach can also lead to concerns about compliance and regulatory knowledge.

Many small private practice physician owners cannot afford a large multi-disciplinary support structure. They must be self-sufficient, knowledgeable of regulations and payment reform models and their impacts to their business. With so much on your plate, it's important to delegate certain tasks to trustworthy staff to allow time for researching, learning and reading. Employ the correct people for the correct jobs to build a solid practice foundation; as they will be an integral part of your ability to provide excellent care.

Usha Sivakumar, MD, Medical Director, Sivimed Internal Medicine and Primary Care Associates.[17]

Staff Training

Human capital is one of an organization's most valuable assets. Employee success starts during the hiring process. Determine practice needs and candidate compatibility prior to hiring. Some hiring managers are willing to train new employees on certain areas of a position. Consider the learning curve and internal support mechanisms when making this decision. Building up staff to be successful will in turn, make the practice successful. Confirm that staff are aware of expectations, responsibilities, and the scope of their position. It's difficult to hold employees accountable for expectations which have either never been or have been poorly communicated to them. Likewise, it is unreasonable to expect an employee to understand the scope of their position or license if it hasn't been reviewed with them. There are many situations in which staff have failed to complete tasks because they lacked understanding of what was expected of them. This can create issues in productivity, employee satisfaction, compliance and patient satisfaction.

Employees should be given a copy of their job description as well as the training and resources required to perform their job adequately. This includes compliance training, role-specific training, development training and more. Regularly meeting with staff allows leadership to provide feedback on performance and expectations by keeping the lines of communication open. Scheduled meetings also allow staff to voice concerns or request additional support. Successful employee relations also include accountability and consequences for poor performance.

Providing tailored training and resources to staff based on position and role is a great way to stay in-tuned with daily operations. This allows leaders to identify gaps in processes and information for resolution. Other corporate training is required to fulfil regulatory compliance requirements.

Biannual HIPAA and Compliance Training

Certified Health Insurance Portability and Accountability Act (HIPAA) programs will review the HIPAA rule and all provisions therein. Staff should review this training annually and test their understanding of HIPAA knowledge. Documentation of all training performed, and all attendees present will support future audits and provide training accountability. Other HIPAA tasks for annual review include things like a review of the HIPAA sanctions policy. This policy reviews the actions to take if the practice identifies a violation of HIPAA policies. HIPAA requires covered entities such as medical practices who store, transmit, and receive protected health information (PHI) to conduct training to ensure its workforce understands the privacy and security measures required to remain compliant. Training a workforce allows a practice to better succeed at keeping patient information private and secure. It is also recommended that practices perform general compliance training with staff for the security of employee records, financial documents, and proprietary practices. Failure to abide by the HIPAA rules and regulations can result in hefty fines and it can also create significant mistrust in patients. Your patients want to know that their information is safe and secure. Many patients have a decent understanding of HIPAA compliance and will recognize when their privacy has been violated. Maintain a strong relationship with your patients and avoid fines by properly training your staff.

> COMPUTER There are many third-party vendors who provide HIPAA training services in-person, online, or via hybrid courses. These solutions can be beneficial to organizations looking for low-cost solutions as opposed to developing internal HIPAA experts. When reviewing external vendors make sure to review their credentials, educational offerings, resources, and policy updates.

At-Hire and Ongoing Job-Specific Training

Employees should understand their role and responsibilities. This means providing new employees with job descriptions, reviewing their productivity, providing ongoing education and training and more. Outlining expectations for employees helps to drive accountability.

Roles should be clear to understand, and training should be role specific. For more information on managing employee roles and responsibilities refer to the Society for Human Resources Management (SHRM) at www.shrm.org or MGMA's Member resources on human resources management.

PCI compliance training

The Payment Card Industry (PCI) Data Security Standard training is specific to credit/debit card handling and processing. As many practices expand on the methods of payments accepted for medical services, it is important for staff to understand requirements for keeping credit card transactions safe. Practices that accept payment cards should perform annual PCI compliance training through their contracted merchant vendor. This regulation is required by the PCI Security Standards Council, which is a "global forum for the ongoing development, enhancement, storage, dissemination and implementation of security standards for account data protection."[18]

Fraud, waste & abuse training (FWA training)

All organizations that accept Medicare Part C & D reimbursements must perform FWA training.[19] FWA training is required by the Department of Health and Human Services (HHS) for all federal healthcare programs and adherence is audited by Office of the Inspector General (OIG) of the HHS. This training is available at CMS.gov.[20] Proof of completion for each employee should be kept in their file. Additional information can be found within the False Claims Act [31 U.S.C. § § 3729-3733] and FWA regulations.

Fair debt collections training (FDCPA)

The Fair Debt Collection Practices Act sets standards for debt collection agencies. While it does not apply to medical practices when seeking to collect on their own debt, any debt collection agency violating these practices would receive significant fines. Although a medical practice is not, under normal circumstances, expected to follow these regulations, billing, front desk, administrative, and collections staff should nonetheless be trained in fair debt collection processes to ensure professionalism and good rapport with patients and the community.

Professional Development

For more comprehensive education, practices can consider structured professional development and/or certification programs. Each career has a starting point. Those of us who are successful have been given the opportunity to learn, grow and expand our knowledge base for personal and professional growth. Practices who place emphasis on professional development have an educated and motivated workforce.

In healthcare, there are many professional certifications that demonstrate one's expertise and mastery of a specific healthcare industry concept. Due to the volume and complexity of concepts, confusing, rapidly changing and even overlapping regulatory standards, many organizations seek to hire certified individuals. This need opens doors for staff to seek additional training and education in an industry that requires subject matter experts.

For practice managers, the key certification is MGMA's American College of Medical Practice Executives (ACMPE) CMPE board certification. This certification verifies that practice administrators have a collegiate-level knowledge in practice administration. It warrants that individuals with the CMPE designation understand the core concepts of revenue cycle management, compliance, human resources, and other critical components of practice management. Each state MGMA has an ACMPE representative who is eager to walk you through the certification process or visit the national MGMA website for more information: www. MGMA.com/acmpe. Individuals interested in obtaining certification in medical record coding may consider the Certified Professional Coder (CPC) designation through AAPC or the Certified Coding Specialist (CCS) designation from AHIMA. There are many other organizations that provide continuing education, resources, and certifications based on health industry topic. Check with the corresponding organization for professional development opportunities.

Having staff pursue certifications and additional industry-specific education helps validate the knowledge level of the employees, fosters learning in best practices, provides opportunities to network with colleagues and clients, and acts as a catalyst for growth in your organization. Additional growth professionally can be achieved through traditional education paths as well. Some organizations offer tuition reimbursement for universities, internal mentorship programs, and paid time off for educational conferences. Maintaining diverse offerings for growth encourages employees to take part in available opportunities.

Oversight

It is not enough to simply train staff and assume they have the behaviors in place to execute accordingly. There should always be an element of oversight to verify that staff are adhering to practice policies.

This can include departmental management (i.e., front desk supervisor, clinical manager, etc.) as well as direct practice manager oversight. Supervisors and managers need to engage with staff to ensure compliance with company policies and to provide updates where needed.

Providing Reference Materials

With ever-changing regulations and policies, it's important to make sure that staff are continuously receiving updates as to what's current. For example, Medicare recently changed the design and layout of their insurance cards, as well as beneficiary IDs.

Practices have been accepting the same type of Medicare card for the last few decades. To suddenly receive a new type of card, with a new design format, and new ID number would be very confusing to the front desk. Failure to go over these changes can lead to delays during check-in, impeding staff efficiency and negatively impact patient experience.

This also applies to annual payer updates. Most insurance companies change some element of their plan ID cards on an annual basis. They may change plan names, group numbers, or standard deductibles and copay amounts. It is a good idea to sign up for payer newsletters for updates.

It's critical that the front desk have a database, or even a notebook, that they can reference that shows some of the current ID cards should look like and where they can find critical information on those cards. For example, they should be able to identify the copay for a specialist or whether a referral is required. Knowing where to identify these on the patient's ID card can save the practice a lot of time during the check in process.

Education on Impactful New Elements

There are regulatory changes that can affect the way practice operates. For example, at the first introduction of sequestration (Medicare payment reductions) in 2013, many practices were caught unaware.[21] Suddenly losing 2% of federal payments for some practices consumed the only margin which existed in their annual budget. (Navigate to Chapter 11 to learn more about sequestration). Another example of regulatory change was the introduction of a penalty for failing to e-prescribe. When this change occurred, there were many practices that had no idea they were taking a penalty for failure to e-prescribe. When billing departments began receiving remittances that documented sequestration and the e-prescribe penalty, there was widespread confusion for those that weren't aware that these policies had changed.

Do not expect the general billing staff or the general front desk staff to individually go out and look for this information. It is the responsibility of management and department supervisors to provide this information to necessary personnel and review on a regular basis.

Engagement

It is also important to have meetings with department staff. Not only to review upcoming changes but, also to review any potential pain points or trends that staff is seeing. For example, staff may start seeing a trend in denied prior authorizations for a regularly used medication. This may prompt the practice manager to reach out to the provider representative for clarification.

Depending on the situation, the providers may need to begin using a different formulary. Alternatively, maybe the providers want to hop on a call with the payer's Chief Medical Officer to clinically understand the reason for denial.

Regardless, this is a situation that can cause significant frustration to patients. Without regular meetings, identification may be too late to prevent a flurry of patient complaints.

✏ Knowledge Check

Practice Preparation

1. **True or False**? Network Adequacy is an audit of provider education which is performed during credentialing

2. EIDM stands for:_____

3. Accounts receivable from a previous PM system may be referred to as _____ A/R.

4. **True or False**? A master project plan should be high-level and doesn't need things like deadlines and contingencies.

5. HIPAA training should take place _____.

6. Methods of connecting to the EHR are often referred to as

   _____.

7. Employees cannot be held accountable for _____ that were never communicated.

Answers:

Q1: False,
Q2: Enterprise Identity Management,
Q3: Legacy,
Q4: False,
Q5: Annually,
Q6: Interfaces,
Q7: Expectations

Endnotes

1. https://www.mgma.com/resources/resources/operations-management/large-group-or-org-practice-startup-checklist

2. Joint Commission International. "Primary Source Verification of Healthcare Professionals; A Risk Reduction Strategy for Patients and Health Care Organizations". https://www.jointcommissioninternational.org/assets/3/7/Risk_Reduction_Strategy_for_Primary_Source_Verification_JCI_2016.pdf

3. CMS Identity & Access Management System: https://nppes.cms.hhs.gov/

4. National Plan & Provider Enumeration System: https://nppes.cms.hhs.gov/

5. CMS: Enterprise Identity Management Overview: https://www.cms.gov/Research-Statistics-Data-and-Systems/CMS-Information-Technology/EnterpriseIdentityManagement/EIDM-Overview.html

6. CMS: Enterprise Identity Management FAQ: https://www.cms.gov/Research-Statistics-Data-and-Systems/CMS-Information-Technology/EnterpriseIdentityManagement/Frequently-Asked-Questions.html

7. NPI Registry: https://npiregistry.cms.hhs.gov/

8. CAQH ProView Application: https://proview.caqh.org

9. CMS Provider Enrollment Revalidation Cycle 2 FAQs: https://www.cms.gov/Medicare/Provider-Enrollment-and-Certification/MedicareProviderSupEnroll/Downloads/Reval_Cycle2_FAQs.pdf

10. https://www.cms.gov/medicare/provider-enrollment-and-certification/medicareprovidersupenroll/revalidations.html

11. CMS: Taxonomy: https://www.cms.gov/Medicare/Provider-Enrollment-and-Certification/MedicareProviderSupEnroll/Taxonomy.html

12. National Uniform Claim Committee http://www.nucc.org/

13. CMS Sample CMS1500: https://www.cms.gov/Medicare/CMS-Forms/CMS-Forms/Downloads/CMS1500.pdf

14. HealthIT.Gov: "Benefits of EHRs" https://www.healthit.gov/topic/health-it-basics/benefits-ehrs

15. Ranges documented by Medical Revenue Cycle Specialists and ITS Healthcare, LLC

16. "Medicare Coordination of Benefits (COB) System Interface Specifications 270/271 Health Care Eligibility Benefit Inquiry and Response HIPAA Guidelines for Electronic Transactions Companion Document for Mandatory Reporting Non-GHP Entities" https://www.cms.gov/Medicare/Coordination-of-Benefits-and-Recovery/Mandatory-Insurer-Reporting-For-Non-Group-Health-Plans/Archive/Downloads/NGHPInterfaceSpecVersion21.pdf

17. Book quote provided by: *Usha Sivakumar, MD, Medical Director, Sivimed Internal Medicine and Primary Care Associates.*

18. https://www.pcisecuritystandards.org/

19. "Medicare Learning Network® (MLN) Medicare Parts C And D Compliance And Fraud, Waste, And Abuse (FWA) Trainings": https://www.cms.gov/Outreach-and-Education/Medicare-Learning-Network-MLN/MLNProducts/Downloads/Fraud-Waste_Abuse-Training_12_13_11.pdf

20. https://www.cms.gov/Outreach-and-Education/Medicare-Learning-Network-MLN/MLNProducts/Downloads/Fraud-Abuse-MLN4649244.pdf

21. CMS Medicare FFS Provider e-News "March 8, 2013": Mandatory Payment Reductions in Medicare Fee-for-Service (FFS) Program – "Sequestration" https://www.cms.gov/Outreach-and-Education/Outreach/FFSProvPartProg/Downloads/2013-03-08-standalone.pdf

Chapter 3

Scheduling & Pre-registration

If a successful RCM program were a fully constructed home, then scheduling and pre-registration would be the foundation. There are a few channels of patient access as it relates to revenue cycle management: (1) during scheduling and pre-registration (2) at the point-of-service, and finally (3) at discharge/check out.

There may be additional opportunities to speak with a patient. There are other reasons for calls between the office and the patient to occur. However, whether these will occur is unknown. Patient access and engagement is important, and by leveraging sound best practices, the practice can contribute to the accuracy and completeness of the patient's account.

Opportunities and Disruptions

Patient access provides opportunities for patient engagement and for potential disruptions to the patient care and RCM processes.

Pre Registration	Obtain individual patient data ahead of the appointment
Patient Scheduling	Schedule the patient for an appointment
Patient Eligibility & Benefits Verification	Verify that the patient's insurance will cover reimbursement for their appointment and educate he patient on their benefits
Authorizations/ Certifications	Verify through the patient's insurance that they are eligible to attend the appointment
Point of Service	Patient arrives for the appointment
Patient Registration	Register the patient into the organization either through paper forms or electronic means
Time of Service Collections	Collect patient balances when they arrive for their appointment
Managing the Waiting Room	Communicate delays with patients, check in patients, and set expectations for wait times
Discharge/ Check-Out	Patient leaves after the appointment

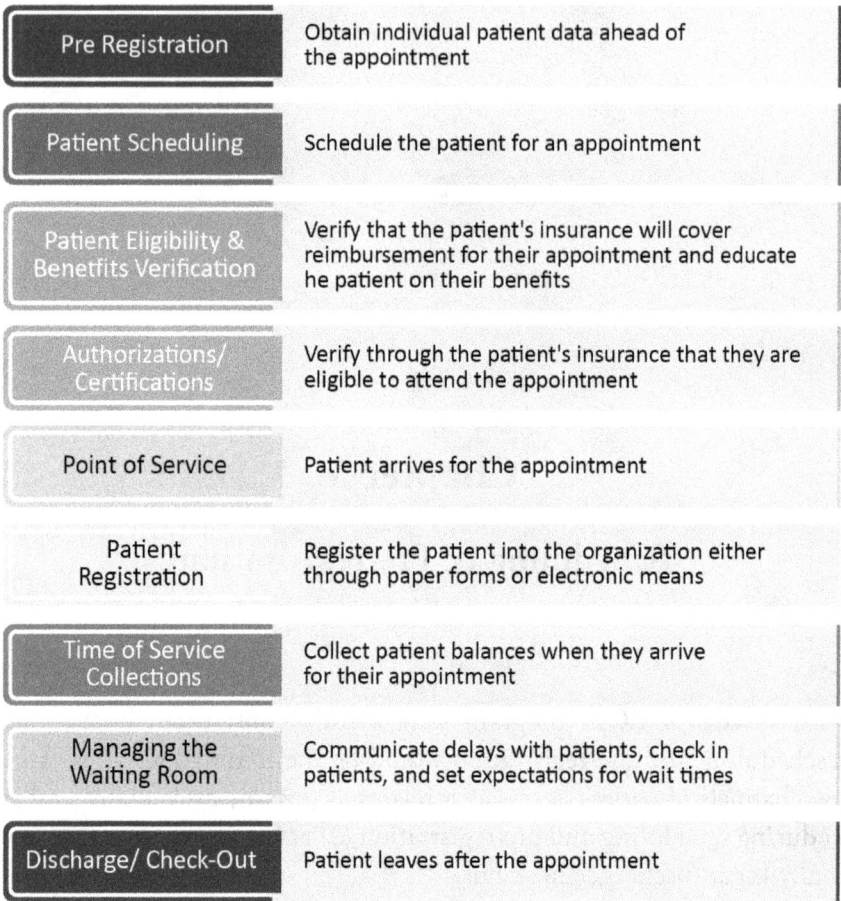

Figure 3.1   Scheduling and pre-registration flow

Patient Scheduling

Good scheduling management allows for efficient office functioning. For example, newborn visits normally include several vaccines. Managing the inventory of vaccines in conjunction with the patient schedule will ensure the vaccines are available for the visit.

The scheduling system chosen must be flexible enough to handle emergency situations, as well as the routine daily schedule. According to Becker's Healthcare's statistics on wait time and patient satisfaction,

"15% of patients wait more than 30 minutes to see a physician. 97% of patients are frustrated by wait times. 80% of respondents said being told the wait time would be either completely or somewhat minimized their frustration."[1]

The ability to schedule efficiently will require attention to the dynamics of the facility:

- **Available resources and staff.** If providers are sharing a medical assistant, then staggering appointment arrival times will help the schedule to stay on track.

- **Time allotted for procedures and testing.** Some appointment types require more time. New patient visits are usually much longer than follow-up visits (depending on complexity) and should regularly require more time.

- **Resource scheduling.** The simultaneous coordination of multiple schedules for the same date of service, i.e., scheduling ultrasound room utilization alongside provider patient schedules. If there is only one ultrasound unit, then patients requiring ultrasound should not be schedule at the same time.

- **Total quantity of exam rooms.** Multiple rooms dedicated to each provider allows for the resetting of one room while the provider is seeing a patient in another room.

- **Proper resource allocation.** When staff have the resources needed to optimize their role in the patient flow, efficiency increases. For example, if there are three medical assistants who bring back patients and they all share one blood pressure cuff, this will cause delays.

SHOUT OUT GUY Proper resource allocation can be a challenge during equipment maintenance. It is essential to thoroughly review vendor contracts and require timely loaner replacements if maintenance is required.

An appointment schedule that accommodates the physician's preferences and commitments allows for smooth operations.

Patient Contact/Call Center

It's common for medical practice resources to be limited. Smaller practices may have staff who wear several hats which may include taking incoming calls and making appointments. For practices that have the bandwidth and have the staffing infrastructure, consider establishing a patient contact center with already existing staff. Practices that need support with answering calls could also benefit from this option. Doing so will optimize the potential of your practice's appointment scheduling system thereby increasing appointment availability, appointment accuracy and meeting quality reporting measures. Using an external patient contact center would augment current practice staff, reducing the volume of incoming requests that current staff must address. Patient calls would route to an internal contact/call center that helps create uniformity in call answering. Contact center staff should be trained in the expectations for communication and documentation. A well-structured contact center will support the proper gathering of pre-registration information and will aid in the decrease of demographic entry errors.

To support your team, provide a reference manual or cheat sheet to any personnel who may answer the phone to support proper process and triage. There are other considerations for successfully integrating a patient contact center into your practice.

> Be mindful not to focus so hard on patient-centric clinical delivery that other communication channels are overlooked. Systems and processes such as patient portals, phone calls to/from patients, appointment reminders, and surveys are all important and require attention. All interactions count when measuring patient satisfaction – not just the face to face ones.
>
> This is particularly true when the size of your business requires a more production-based environment and many front-

desk functions such as communicating lab results, adjusting appointment dates/times, and answering questions on medications as an example, are managed through a contact center structure. Patient contact centers are the most effective way to efficiently manage large volumes of patient and partner contacts, but they should be designed in such a way as to honor and protect the sanctity of the provider-patient relationship. Remember that your business is only as strong as its weakest link.

Contact centers also provide opportunities to more easily view trends, capture valuable reporting data, reduce overall operating costs, and maximize opportunities to generate revenues. One example is to leverage contact center capabilities to run campaigns for Annual Wellness Visit (AWV) reminders, support Chronic Care Management (CCM) programs for remote patient care, and provide 24x7 nurse lines in-center or in a work from home setting.[2]

Larry Hefling, Owner at ITS Strategic Consulting, LLC

SHOUT OUT GUY To minimize risk in the organization ensure the call center workflows route clinical calls directly to clinical personnel.

Scheduling Instructions

Your front desk needs guidance. Providers and management should provide instructions for appointment scheduling, set forth in writing, and clearly communicated to the scheduling staff.

Best Practices

Schedule optimization occurs with the implementation of best practices. These best practices include scheduling lookbacks to review historical scheduling data and identify opportunities to improve. This process may identify regulatory changes or insurance payer changes. Periodic updates to policies and procedures of external entities are important to review because they may affect the scheduling process. For example, if a payer changes a reimbursement policy of a surgical procedure and now requires a prior authorization that will change the timeline for scheduling the procedure.

This industry has frequently changing regulations. Structured change management processes will help to prepare for these changes, to ensure smooth transitions across the organization and to provide comprehensive staff education and training. These processes should include documenting changes to workflows and staff requirements, updating reference documents, disseminating to the team, and providing opportunities for staff to ask questions.

> In the business of healthcare, revenue cycle management is critical as reimbursements continue to decline and costs of doing business continue to increase. Revenue cycle management starts at the front desk with staff appropriately trained to obtain correct billing and demographic information as well as to perform benefit verifications. Accuracy in registration and data collection creates a seamless and streamlined process for claims to be submitted in order for reimbursements to be received. Without correct front desk data collection, claims can be denied, timely filing deadlines missed, and revenues lost. Well-trained front desk staff become extremely important to the success of any medical practice.[3] *Alta Sharp, Sharp Physician Services*

Standardization

Providers have standing orders and operating procedures for a reason. They set expectations and allow for greater efficiency. For this reason, each scheduled procedure should have a standard appointment length that is built into the system to maximize scheduling.

There will be situations that require an override of pre-set appointment times. For example, a provider may want more time for an appointment with a particularly complex patient. Select supervisors should have instructions and authority to override. These individuals can communicate scheduling needs and understand the overall workflow of the providers.

New Patient Visits

An individual should be considered a "new patient" if they have not been seen by any provider in the practice in the last three years. Patients who are new to a practice will need to provide key pieces of information for healthcare service delivery, consent to treatments and payment for services.

All new patients require pre-registration via telephone or in person when scheduling their appointment. New patient packets, mailed or on a practice website, can be very useful in obtaining preliminary patient demographics information. New patient packets often include items like practice brochures, no-show policy, a financial policy, and new patient registration forms. It is a good practice to register new patients at least 24 hours prior to visit. For same day visits, registration occurs upon check in.

> SHOUT OUT GUY   Even with proper precautions, delays will occur, and schedules will periodically fall behind. Apprising patients of delays allows the patient the option of rescheduling their appointment if desired. Clear and proactive communication will prevent most patients from minding the wait.

Scripting

Practices should create a written script for staff, but they should be encouraged to personalize the standard scripting. The script should assist the collection of all pertinent patient information during scheduling.

Pre-registration

Pre-registration is one step that practices skip because the sense is that they "don't have time" or "don't have staff" to complete. Pre-registration is an important service that benefits the clinical workflow as well as revenue cycle management and saves time at check-in, enabling the practice to verify patient eligibility and benefits prior to the visit. This process requires both time and staff.

Sixty-one percent of initial denials are due to demographic/technical errors, followed by eligibility 16% and medical necessity 12%. Forty-two percent of denial write-offs are due to demographic/technical errors.[4]

Pre-registration Review

Pre-registration review includes looking for missing patient demographics, verifying insurance, conducting benefit eligibility and contacting the patient to verify and combine with the reminder call where appropriate. During the pre-registration process can confirm, at a minimum, patient demographics (see Appendix A) and insurance information (insurer, plan type, member ID, copay, policy holder).

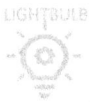

> Proper pre-registration reduces daily call volume and enhances patient-to-practice communications. Auditing quality, scoring, and educating staff toward improvement can also reduce daily call volume and enhance patient-to-practice communications.

Additional items to discuss with the patient include:

- Arrival time and if patients should come early or with additional forms completed (new patient forms, new problem forms, etc.).
- Any additional information patients should bring to their appointment (medication lists, referrals, etc.).
- Expectations of copays or outstanding balances at the time of service.

- Notification to patients that appointments will be self-pay if no insurance is given or verification of insurance coverage fails.

Insurance Verification is the process by which the practice personnel verify a patient's insurance eligibility and benefits for prospective visits, procedures, and/or testing. Verification is not a confirmation of payment but is instead a confirmation that the patient does have insurance coverage and payment is possible.

Insurance verification

This is one of, if not *the* most important foundational blocks of your RCM process.

It is not possible to achieve consistent RCM success without this step.

This includes a thorough evaluation with the insurer, either on the phone or through an electronic verification portal. During the evaluation:

1. Confirm the right patient is being reviewed.

2. Make sure to review the service level, coinsurance, copays, and deductibles.

3. Document the subscriber of the insurance and whether the patient is a dependent.

4. Document the effective dates of the insurance benefits.

5. Identify if referrals are required.

6. Identify in-network and out-of-network benefits.

7. Confirm the patient's address and the insurance plan name.

> SHOUT OUT GUY
> An analysis of 3.3 billion hospital transactions in 2016 by *Becker's Hospital Review* found registration/eligibility (23.9%) of insurance denials.[5]

Required Competency Standards for Staff Performing Verifications

Performing eligibility verifications is a critical component of the RCM process and, as such, personnel should have proper training. See Appendix I for more information on competency standards for these individuals.

Scheduling Best Practices

Patient appointment scheduling is a necessary component of patient care and initiation of the revenue cycle. Information collected during scheduling directly contributes to the claim's submission process. For this reason, it's important to establish best practices that support accurate and timely collection of data and scheduling documentation. The process of best practices in scheduling include:

Early verifications. Demographic and insurance information collected are verified prior to or at the time of the appointment.

100% registration. Patient registration in the PM system for the purposes of billing, contracting, and data analysis.

New, difficult, and complex patients. New, difficult, and complex patients should not be double-booked. *Double-booking* is when two appointments are scheduled in the same time slot. This sometimes happens due to overflow or blocking similar services together. Double-booking is problematic for new patients, though, because the time required for new patients (and established patients with new problems) is unpredictable. Consecutive new patients, difficult patients, or patients with complex conditions can also create difficulty in the schedule.

Comprehensive documentation. Basic information to document and store includes full patient demographics (see Appendix A for more information). Guarantor data must also be collected for patient statements and payment collection when the patient is not the responsible party for payment.

If applicable, documented approvals may provide (secure and encrypted) patient information or payment information through the practice website or patient portal. Staff collection and entry of all required and pertinent patient information collected to thoroughly completes the patient's demographic account.

New Patients

The steps below outline an example process for onboarding new patients.

Complete demographic form

Demographic forms in an organization are either paper or electronic and provide a standardized method of capturing crucial patient information. This form should include the basic data required to input the patient into the practice EHR. Please see Appendix for a sample patient registration form. Practices that have abolished the use of a patient registration form, will complete pre-registration through the use of EHR and validate this information when the patient presents for an office visit.

Scan Front and Back of Insurance Card

Most EHRs have a method to scan in the patient's insurance card. This information is extremely helpful to the revenue cycle process and can be a critical element when working claim denials. It is essential to enter the patient's information *exactly* as listed on the insurance card. If there is an error on the patient's insurance card, the patient will need to address that with the insurer directly. Entering the patient's name into the practice management system in a way that doesn't match their insurance card will likely result in claims denials.

Scan Patient's or Responsible Party's Driver's License

Scanning the patient or responsible party's identification provides a method to visually confirm the patient in the future, while also meeting a red flag measure (see Chapter 16). Some EHRs have the capability to store a patient's photo in their chart. This is another excellent identification method and should be implemented where available.

Some steps to take if the name on the driver's license does not match the insurance card:

- If it is a typo on the insurance card, instruct the patient to contact their insurance company to update their information. The contact phone number should be on the back of their insurance card.
- If it is completely different, ask the patient if the name on the insurance card is the subscriber.
- Request another form of identification to match with insurance information.
- Ask individual to state secured information that only the patient should have access to, such as, asking them to state the patient's Social Security number or patient portal password.
- If staff is concerned that an individual is falsely using someone else's insurance information, train them to discreetly contact a manager. The manager will further assess the situation and either confirm the patient's identity or contact local police if the identity appears to be fraudulent.

Confirm Copay or Co-insurance

Except for preventive services, most visits will have a copay amount due. It is a good idea to confirm the amount due prior to the patient's appointment for collection during checking. For more information on understanding patient copays and coinsurances, refer to the section below on "Understanding Patient Insurance Cards."

Complete Patient History Forms, If Applicable

Require staff collect and document a patient's personal, familial, and social histories. This is essential to the providers during treatment and obtaining this information for all new patients sets a baseline for future updates.

> COMPUTER The practice can employ technology for gathering patient check-in information. Patients can enter demographic data into a tablet or through a patient portal and save a step for the front desk, who will now have this information at their fingertips.

Review the Form for Completeness and Signatures.

While you have face-to-face access to the patient, verify that the forms are complete and obtain any required signatures (consent to treat, consent to text, etc.).

In order to set national standards for the protection of protected health information, the Health Insurance Portability and Accountability Act of 1996 (HIPAA), was enacted by the U.S. Congress and signed into law by President Bill Clinton. In fulfilling HIPAA compliance requirements, adherence to the Security Rule and the Privacy Rule is paramount. The Security Rule established national standards to protect individuals' electronic personal health information (ePHI) by requiring administrative, physical and technical safeguards to ensure the confidentiality, integrity, and security of ePHI. Whereas, the Privacy Rule requires safeguards to protect the privacy of personal health information and sets limits and conditions on the uses and disclosures and mandates some disclosures cannot be made without patient authorization. The Rule includes a set of patient's rights about how to access their health information, including rights to examine and obtain a copy of health records, and to request corrections. Together, both Rules set the foundation and specifications for how healthcare organizations must implement a security management process to secure and safeguard protected health information and how to administer a comprehensive HIPAA compliance program.[6]

Jay Hodes, President of Colington Consulting

> SHOUT OUT GUY   Research into federal regulations, state regulations, and specialty requirements on consent documentation can prove beneficial. For example, you are required to obtain patient consent before texting protected information or leaving a detailed voicemail with protected information. Staff education on HIPAA rules and other regulations that protect patient information is vital.

Established Patient

An individual is an *established* or *existing patient* if they have been seen by a provider within the practice in the last three years. The steps below outline an example process for properly maintaining the information the practice has for established patients.

Confirm Demographic Information

Demographic information should be confirmed at least annually. Review the basic demographic information with the patient to document updates. Focus areas include the address, phone number, insurance carrier, member ID, insurance subscriber, group number, and copay.

Confirm Insurance Information

To help confirm insurance information, scan the front and back of the patient's insurance card at least annually into the EHR or PM system.

Most visits will have a copayment amount due. Always confirm the amount due prior to the patient's appointment for collection during check in. For more information on understanding patient insurance information, refer to the section below on "Understanding Patient Insurance Cards."

If your practice is still using paper processes, make a copy of the patient's insurance card, front and back, to retain with the patient chart.

COMPUTER If your PM or EHR system allows the scanning and retention of patient ID cards; you should take advantage of this capability. If you wait to identify incorrect entries after claims submission, then the patient is no longer on site and access to the information is much harder to obtain. Scanned insurance cards can also help to support the appeals process for denied claims and scanned insurance cards are usually more legible than copied insurance cards.

Complete Patient History Forms

When applicable, patient history forms should be updated regularly. Sometimes these updates happen at the front desk; in other instances, they occur in the exam room during intake. This will vary based on workflow. Complete and up-to-date forms support the coding process and can provide justification for the level of CPT® selected.

Understanding Patient Insurance Cards

Member's name. Confirm accuracy of spelling of member's name. There are instances in which an insurance company has a member's name listed differently than their government issued ID or than what the practice has on file. In some situations, this will not be the name of your patient. Some insurers will list the names of the dependents, others will issue cards to each dependent, and others will only have one card that only lists the name of the subscriber.

It is beneficial to confirm with the patient. Submit claims using the exact information found on the insurance card. Doing so will ensure that the insurance company can identify the member in their database. If corrections are required, work with the patient to update insurance records.

Member ID number. This number is critical for insurance verification and claims payment. Careful input of this number and confirmation of accuracy is important before moving forward.

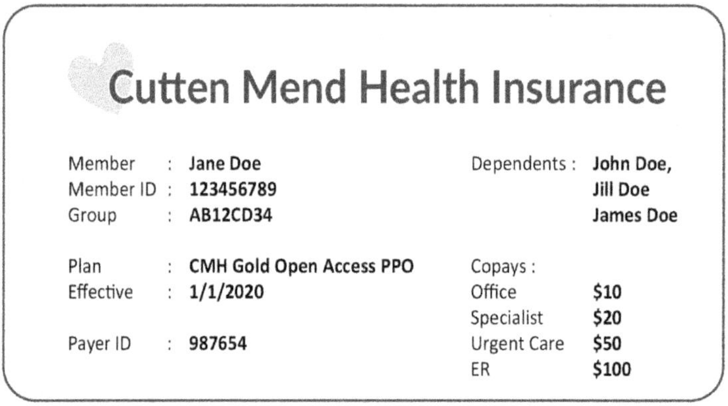

Cutten Mend Health Insurance			
Member	: Jane Doe	Dependents :	John Doe,
Member ID	: 123456789		Jill Doe
Group	: AB12CD34		James Doe
Plan	: CMH Gold Open Access PPO	Copays :	
Effective	: 1/1/2020	Office	$10
		Specialist	$20
Payer ID	: 987654	Urgent Care	$50
		ER	$100

Figure 3.2   Sample insurance card – front view

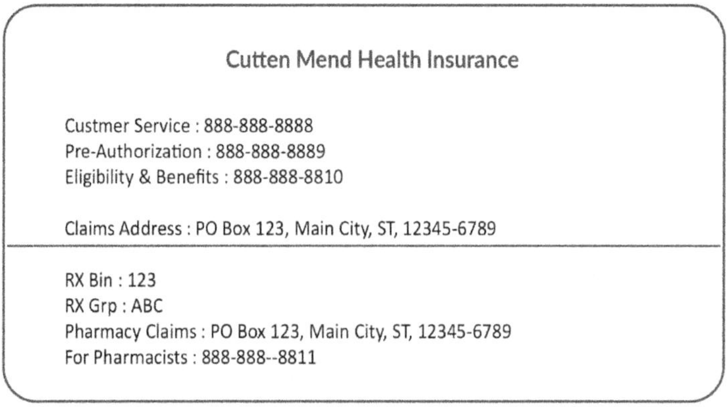

Cutten Mend Health Insurance

Custmer Service : 888-888-8888
Pre-Authorization : 888-888-8889
Eligibility & Benefits : 888-888-8810

Claims Address : PO Box 123, Main City, ST, 12345-6789

RX Bin : 123
RX Grp : ABC
Pharmacy Claims : PO Box 123, Main City, ST, 12345-6789
For Pharmacists : 888-888--8811

Figure 3.3   Sample insurance card – back view

Group number. This number is usually associated with the subscriber's employer group or plan administrator and is a required data field for claims processing and benefits verification. This number identifies the employer to the insurance payer. Errors in this field will result in claim denials.

Copays. The category and copay type varies by practice, provider, and service type but should be communicated to the front desk for proper payment collection. Often cards will reflect different amounts for urgent care and specialists as well as those listed above.

Annual visits, preventive services, and certain testing will not have a copay and collecting one for these types of services may result in additional work. For example, collecting a copay for an annual wellness visit will result in extra work for the back office and will generate a task to issue a patient refund. This is another reason why verifying copays prior to each appointment is essential.

> SHOUT OUT GUY   Reference guides at the front desk with example images of insurance cards for payers in your area can be very helpful. This is especially true when the reference guide is notated with key identification points and participation status. Other pertinent notations in this guide like "referrals required" or "referring provider name required" can empower the front desk to be as accurate as possible.

Other key data elements to consider when reviewing an insurance card include:

Primary care provider (PCP). If your practice is providing primary care services and your provider's name is not listed on the patient's insurance card as required, your claims will most likely be denied. Have the patient change assigned PCP's prior to providing care.

In-Network deductible and coinsurance. If this information is stated on the card, call to determine how much of the deductible is met. This will let you know the likelihood of your claims being unpaid, especially for high deductible plans.

Out-of-Network deductible and coinsurance. In the event your provider is not participating with a patient's insurance, it's important to check this benefit to determine coverage and out-of-pocket expenses.

Plan contact information. Always confirm the plan claims address and phone number.

Denials based upon issues with registration information (i.e., incorrect name spelling, missing PCP on insurance card, incorrect subscriber, etc.) can be very difficult to overturn or to win on appeal. For this reason, it is beneficial to confirm the accuracy of this information before the patient's visit. Shown below is an example of a claim denial due to missing PCP information.

Patient Provider	DOS	Proc	Mod	Billed	Allowed	Pt. Resp	Paid	Remark
John Doe Dr. Smitha	1/1/2021	99213		100.00	00	00	00	
	1/1/2021	96372	25	25.00	00	00	00	
			Total	125.00	00	00	00	

Cutten Mend Health Insurance
Explanation of Benefits

Remark Codes : **N778 Missing primary care physician information**

Payment: **CHECK**
Tracking#: **123456**
Date: **1/31/2021**

Figure 3.4   Example claim denial

Revitalizing the Patient Interview Process

Now that you know what you need to do, you may be wondering how to get this information from the patient. You will want to avoid any obstacles to obtaining the information that is needed. It is recommended that you physically review a patient's insurance card at every visit. This may seem redundant but staying vigilant about data accuracy is key. After a while, patients will come to expect this process from your practice and see it as your dedication to accuracy. This theme should follow through to treatment.

To gain patient's buy-in to processes, it's best to start with education. When asking for insurance information, consider making conversation about how tricky insurance can be and your office's goal to get it right the first time to avoid any unnecessary bills.

During the verification process patients should present their picture ID. This process verifies patient identity just as a retail location would do when processing a credit card, and it may help to relay that to the patient to provide context.

Collecting money from sick people isn't a glamourous job. Who really wants to ask someone who isn't feeling well for money? In order to stay in business, provide excellent care, and adhere to insurance participation agreements, practices must follow through with this task. Notifying patients of their financial responsibilities during interactions such as at scheduling, during pre-registration, after insurance verification, within appointment confirmations and reminders is beneficial.

It's always best to give patients a heads up about monies owed before they present for an appointment; no one wants to be blindsided with an unexpected request for payment.

Good Patient Interview Questions vs. Bad Patient Interview Questions

It can be fascinating to observe how asking a poorly-worded question will deliver the wrong information or prime the patient to respond in a way that is not useful, while a well-worded question will prime them to readily understand what is needed and deliver what will be useful.

The below table has a comparison of the sorts of answers bad or good questions will evoke in the pursuit of patient encounter goals.

Goal	Bad Questions	Wrong Answers	Good Questions	Right Answers
To confirm up-to-date insurance information	Has anything changed?	No.	Do you still have Cutten Mend Health Insurance?	No, I almost forgot, thank you for saying that, we changed to Big Federal in January.
To confirm address, phone, etc.	Any changes to your contact info?	No.	Are you still located on Happy Valley Lane?	Oh my, no we moved last June, I thought my husband called in.
Resolving patient communication issues	You aren't getting our invoices? I will let billing know.	No opportunity to answer.	You aren't getting our invoices? Let's go through what we have in our system. Do you still live at 1234 Madison?	Oh, that's it! No, we moved.
Collecting patient copays	You have a $20 copay. Should we bill you?	Yes, please. Thank you!	Your copay is $20. Will that be cash or card?	Cash please. Thank you!

Goal	Bad Questions	Wrong Answers	Good Questions	Right Answers
Collecting past due balances	Did you know you have a balance?	Yes. Thanks, I know. I'll take care of it later… when I hit the lottery.	I see that our billing staff has spoken with you about your outstanding balance. I can collect that $50 from you now. Will that be cash or card?	Card please.
Increasing patient portal use	Did you know that we have a patient portal?	Yup, I'm not interested. Thanks.	I can go ahead and get you registered with our patient portal, so next time you can complete your paperwork online and show up at your appointment time instead of twenty minutes early.	You mean I can sleep in instead of hanging out in the waiting room? Sign me up!

✎ Chapter 3 Knowledge Check

Scheduling & Pre-registration

Question #1:

_____ A term for money collected while the patient is in the office to be seen.

Question #2:

The information needed to verify patient's insurance can be found on

_____

Question #3:

Most patient visits have what type of payment due?_____

Question #4:

True or False? It is recommended to review patient insurance cards at every visit.

Answers:

Q1: Time-Of-Service Collections
Q2: The Patient's Insurance Card
Q3: A Copayment Amount

Q4: True

Endnotes

1. Becker's Hospital Review: "9 Statistics on Wait Times and Patient Satisfaction." 12/20/2013. https://www.beckershospitalreview.com/quality/9-statistics-on-wait-times-and-patient-satisfaction.html

2. Book quote provided by: Larry Hefling, Owner at ITS Strategic Consulting, LLC

3. Book quote provided by: Alta Sharp, Sharp Physician Services

4. Becker's Hospital Review, "4 ways healthcare organizations can reduce claim denials" https://www.beckershospitalreview.com/finance/4-ways-healthcare-organizations-can-reduce-claim-denials.html

5. Becker's Hospital Review "Denial rework costs providers roughly $118 per claim: 4 takeaways https://www.beckershospitalreview.com/finance/denial-rework-costs-providers-roughly-118-per-claim-4-takeaways.html

6. Book quote provided by: Jay Hodes, President of Colington Consulting

Chapter 4

Eligibility, Referrals, & Authorizations

Patient Eligibility and Benefits

The process of checking patient eligibility and benefits is one of the most significant portions of the RCM process. The accuracy of the information directly impacts the speed of reimbursement and whether the insurer will reimburse future claims. This information is also connected to the patient's profile that is used for a host of various purposes. For example, in addition to billing activities, patient contact information is also used to provide test results and make follow up appointments. Incorrect information that is entered into a system and remains on file for a patient could impact the quality of care.

It is important to verify insurance eligibility for every date-of-service (DOS) because patient's insurance coverage may change mid-year for many reasons:

Changes in employment or spouse's employment. When patients or their spouses change employment, they may experience a change in insurance coverage from one carrier to another or even from one plan to another within the same carrier.

Failure to pay insurance premiums. There are policies on the marketplace that patients can come on and off monthly depending on whether they've made their premium payments.

Mid-year renewal cycles. Not all insurance policies renew January 1st of a year. Many renew at other times throughout the year in alignment with a different fiscal cycle or for some other reason. During renewals, subscribers may choose different carriers and plans.

Change in benefit coordination. If a patient no longer has multiple policies, then a formerly secondary policy may now be primary. Alternatively, perhaps the patient has historically had only Medicare, but now, their spouse is working full-time and covering them as a dependent under their employer-group health plan. In either situation, the order to bill insurance changed, impacting the process of claims submission. There are many other situations that can prompt a change in benefit coordination as well.

Aging out of parental plans. Children can remain on their parents' insurance plans much longer now, but there are still set parameters for when they will "age out." This means they've grown too old for their parents to cover them as dependents. In these situations, patients may obtain coverage through their employer, their spouse, their school, or the HIE.

Medicaid MCOs. Some MCOs allow the patient to change plans monthly. Not verifying insurance could result in submitting claims to the wrong payer.

High-deductible plans. The cost of care is not declining, which results in employers being forced to control costs by selecting high deductible plans. These plans require a higher out-of-pocket expense for the patient. In order to understand the patient's benefits for the date of service, specialty, and services provided, it's important to verify insurance to attempt to determine the status of a patient's unmet deductible. This provides an indication to the practice that there may be an out-of-pocket responsibility to collect up front. This may also be an indication that a patient may require a payment plan before moving forward with additional procedures.

Conveniently, most practice management systems allow for electronic eligibility and benefits verification, and for those that don't, there are web portals and insurance phone lines dedicated to supporting this task.

COMPUTER   If you aren't sure how to access this information in your system, contact your EHR or PM vendor. If you do not have access to do this electronically through your system, navigate to the insurers website (listed on the patient's card) to verify benefits. If you are not able to login to the payer's website, call the phone number on the back of the insurance card to verify.

Fundamental Information for the Verification Process

Patient demographics. Patient's name, address, and ID number, as documented on their paperwork, must match what the payer has on file. For a full list of patient demographics, refer to Appendix A.

Eligibility dates. This refers to the dates the patient has coverage. The prospective DOS must be within that timeframe to be reimbursed by the insurance payer. Sometimes a patient has a future date for coverage to begin and any services prior to that date will be denied.

Type of insurance. The insurance type will guide whether the patient requires a referral. There are many types of insurance plans including two very common types of insurance: Health Maintenance Organizations (HMOs) and Preferred Provider Organizations (PPOs). For a full list of insurance types with descriptions, see Chapter 6.

Patient Responsibilities

The responsibilities of the patient are amounts they or their guarantor have financial responsibility, including the patient's deductible, coinsurance, copay and coverages.

Deductible

This is a preset amount that the insurance company requires a patient to pay before the insurer will reimburse the physician directly for any services rendered. Many insurance plans that include a deductible may also have a lower premium amount. Some employers who offer a group health plan, may provide its employees (your patients) with a fixed amount of payroll deducted financial assistance with insurance premium payments. The deductible amount is in addition to the insurance premium. With the rising costs of healthcare, deductible amounts are trending upward, leaving many patients with higher out of pocket expenses.

For example, a patient may pay $300 per month in premiums for participation with XYZ Insurance and may still need to pay $1,000.00 out-of-pocket expenses before the insurer will reimburse the physician for any services rendered. Since some physician services will not be paid until after a deductible is met, it's important to determine a patient's deductible amount, how much of it has been met and the amount remaining patient's out of pocket expense prior to services being rendered. Some plans may have individual and family deductibles. Deductible information may be obtained during the insurance verification process.

Coinsurance

Some insurance plans include required coinsurance amounts due from the patient for each service rendered. The coinsurance is the out-of-pocket amount that the patient must pay after the deductible is met. Yes, there are more out-of-pocket expenses for your patients! The coinsurance amount doesn't kick in until after the deductible has been met.

Again, in order to determine a patient's out-of-pocket expenses, verify insurance and ask the representative to provide you with the patient's deductible amount, whether there is an individual or family deductible, how much of the deductible is met, and, once it's met, the amount of the patient's coinsurance.

For example, if an insurer is reimbursing a physician $100 for a service, but the patient has a 20% coinsurance after the deductible is met, then the insurer will pay $80 and the remaining $20 will be due from the patient to the provider. It will be the responsibility of the practice to collect this payment amount, so it is beneficial to discuss these benefits and amounts with the patient prior to services being rendered.

Premium	Deductible	Coinsurance
Amount paid monthly to the insurer to keep benefits active.	Used to decrease or offset insurance premium costs.	The out of pocket amount that the patient must pay after the deductible is met.
For employer group plans, this is usually a payroll deduction from the employee/subscriber's paycheck.	Patient is responsible for paying this amount before payments will be made to their healthcare providers.	Due from the patient to the practice, this doesn't kick in until after the deductible has been met.

Figure 4.1   Premium, deductible, and coinsurance information

Some practices may or may not choose to collect deductibles and coinsurances after the claim has been adjudicated by the payer. A few factors to consider when deciding when to collect deductibles and coinsurance include:

1. Has the patient received any other medical services that are still in the adjudication process by the insurance that have not been applied to the deductible? This will impact the amount of the remaining deductible if other healthcare services have not been applied prior to the date of service that you are treating the patient.

2. Does the patient have an individual or family deductible and, if so, which one must be met for a coinsurance to kick in? If the full family deductible must be met, then that will take more time, as family deductibles are higher than individual deductibles. Usually, the individual deductible must be met for reimbursement of services to occur.

3. Where is the benefits and insurance information coming from? Your reimbursement is only as good as the data that is given to you. Some PM software or clearinghouses may not have real-time claims adjudication information. Consider reaching out to the insurance directly for this information.

Copayment

Many insurance types and plans include a copay amount due at the DOS payable to the practice from the patient. These amounts can vary depending on specialty. This amount is agreed upon by the insurance and the patient. As part of the practice's participation contract with the payer, the practice agrees to collect the copay at the time of service. With the rise of preventive care measures, some plans will waive the copayment for benefit-approved preventive services.

For example, a patient may need to pay $30 for an office visit with their PCP or $60 to see a specialist. For some plans, there are also separate copay amounts for hospital and urgent care visits. Always collect copays on the DOS at check-in.

Coverage

With all the various coverage options, each employer or benefit group has the choice to select the coverage that they prefer. A teacher's union may have different coverage than an IT company. Although it's in the patient's best interest to understand their coverage, that is not always the case, so the practice must educate its staff and patients. A review of the patient's coverage will identify if the services require referral or authorization, will confirm non-covered services and, in some situations, will prompt the organization to complete an Advance Beneficiary Notice (ABN).

Advance Beneficiary Notice (ABN)

An ABN is a notification to patients that their insurance will not cover a prospective procedure. The notification includes the expected out-of-pocket expense for the patient along with the procedure description. When a provider finds that a service is medically necessary but may not be a covered benefit for their patient under their insurance plan, they use an ABN.

ABNs are a requirement whenever it is known that a procedure will not be covered. For example, if a patient's insurance benefits do not cover allergy shots, but the patient wants them anyway, an ABN must be on file to legally bill the patient.

Each insurance payer may have specific requirements for example, below are Medicare's requirements:[1]

Please do the following when you want to have a beneficiary sign an ABN.

- Review the ABN with the beneficiary or his/her representative and answer any questions before they sign the form
- The ABN must be delivered far enough in advance that the beneficiary or representative has time to consider the options and make an informed choice
- Once all blanks are completed and the form is signed, a copy is given to the beneficiary or representative
- In all cases, the notifier must retain the original notice on file

Note: Employees or subcontractors of the notifier may deliver the ABN. ABNs are never required in emergency or urgent care situations.

There should be an area for the patient's signature on the ABN. The original should go into the patient record and a copy should go to the patient. There are instances when a patient will submit notification to the insurer that a practice is "errantly billing" them for uncovered services. To clear any misunderstandings with the payer, it is critical that the ABN be accurate, signed, and available to the billing staff.

The ABN should explain to the patient that although their insurance may not cover a service, the healthcare provider would like to move forward because, in their clinical opinion, the service is medically necessary. Additionally, since the patient's insurance may not cover the service, the ABN is signed as an indicator that the patient understands these factors and agrees to be financially responsible for the non-covered service. Without an ABN, in most cases, a provider is prohibited from billing a patient for a non-covered service. The ABN allows the provider to bill the patient outside of their benefits for the non-covered service.

Documenting the completed ABN in one standard place is critical so that the billing staff and any other individuals who participate in the RCM process can locate this information for verification as needed. Have a process that outlines where to document or refer to this information and educate staff accordingly.

Routine Use of ABNs

Although you may be tempted to standardize your workflows by pre-empting denials for services you believe might be denied, CMS prohibits routine use of ABNs.

> A notice given out on a routine basis, which does no more than state Medicare payment denial is possible, is not an acceptable advance notice. We do not accept statements like, 'I never know if Medicare will deny payment,' and similar generalizations for advance notice purposes.[2]

Examples of potential ABN misuse:

- Including a generic ABN in a standard new patient packet for all patients to complete regardless of patient's insurance coverage and benefits.
- Consistently having patients complete ABNs for a specific procedure, regardless of patient's insurance coverage and benefits.

If you aren't sure whether your process is appropriate, keep this in mind: this is a protocol for when providers deem a service medically necessary and it is *not* covered by the patient's insurance. Therefore, if you are attempting to complete ABNs before verifying insurance and benefits, it is likely an inappropriate usage.

SHOUT OUT GUY The use of ABNs is really triggered by the provider's knowledge of the payer's coverage for a service and the provider's belief in the medical necessity for that uncovered service. Do you have a process for educating providers or do you provide quick-reference guides to support providers in identifying when ABNs are necessary? One way of determining whether a service is covered or not is by searching the Medicare Physician Fee: if there is no allowable amount, this is an indication that an ABN may be required. If you are building a reference guide for your providers, consider listing frequently performed procedures along with most frequently billed insurances. Cross reference this information to determine what services are not covered by each plan to create a process for obtaining ABNs from your patients.

Referrals and Authorizations

Referrals and authorizations are large contributors to the success of the RCM, but they are not interchangeable terms. They each represent similar but different components of the RCM. Failure to manage these elements may result in significant and negative impacts to the revenue cycle. Of note, most provider insurance participation agreements prohibit the provider from billing a patient if a service is denied for no referral or authorization.

Referrals

Referrals permit a patient to see a different provider. For example, a PCP may refer a patient with diabetes to see an endocrinologist. If the patient has an HMO, it will likely require a referral to the endocrinologist directly from their PCP. If the patient arrives without a referral, this can create a problem for the endocrinologist, as submission without a referral may not guarantee payment. Referrals are usually *not* required for patients with an open access plan. The patient's insurance card should identify referral requirements for specialists. Additionally, this information is available during benefit verification.

In general, referrals include the type of prospective treatment, how many visits are authorized, and when the referral expires. Different insurance companies may have different requirements for referrals. For example, some may require that referrals expire within six months, while others may require that referrals just expire within the year. Some referrals may list no more than three visits per referral, while others may list ninety-nine.

It is critical, prior to scheduling appointments that the front desk staff identify if the patient has any open referrals. Patients with referral requirements must have an open referral prior to appointment. Referrals should be present no later than 48-hours prior to appointment, otherwise, the practice is at risk of not collecting reimbursement for that visit.

Develop an Effective Referral Plan

Developing an effective referral plan is much like developing an effective authorization plan. Identifying frequent referring providers allows for an open communication process to collaboratively manage the referral process. Educating patients on referral responsibilities during appointment scheduling gives them an opportunity to request required referrals prior to visits. In most payer participation agreements, insurance companies will inform healthcare providers that they may not bill a member if the provider fails to obtain a required referral. Patients should be made aware of all services that require a referral prior to services being rendered. Create a practice policy that adheres to your payer participation agreements regarding the how you address services that require referrals and patient responsibilities.

Develop a consistent identification method. A set process for checking the benefits and requirement of each patient's plan effects the entire revenue cycle, not just the referral process.

Document the referral process. Reference manuals which document processes give your staff guidance on how to request and confirm referrals. Additionally, this documentation provides expectations for staff whether new or existing.

Plan for ongoing staff education. As insurance plans change their requirements, notify the front desk. Usually the billing manager is accountable to perform this education. Make it a known part of the referral management process.

Develop a system that monitors status of referrals. Electronic records systems will often countdown the number of remaining referrals. Each system requires a different process, verify with your IT support or EHR rep. For those on paper charts, file referrals in the patient chart and document dates of usage. When referrals have been exhausted, contact the patient or their PCP for a new referral as needed.

Have a documented plan for issue management. If a patient presents without a referral what are the next steps for the front desk? Should the staff immediately reach out to the PCP for a new referral? Should they immediately reschedule the patient? These policies require agreement at the leadership level, documentation and distribution to all staff.

Document referrals

Referrals can be maintained with the patient chart or in the PM system to attach to claims as needed. Refer to Chapter 5, for an example.

COMPUTER Utilize your EHR to count down the number of visits remaining on a referral. If the original referral has 3 visits, create a tracker that deducts visits from that original count so that you can request a new referral prior to the visits running out. Include the patient in obtaining a new referral prior to expiration of visits. Keep track of payer referral visit maximums.

Authorizations

The authorization process is the path by which a patient's insurer determines if they will reimburse the provider for a future procedure. If a payer requires authorization for a procedure, then failure to obtain one will result in a denial of payment.

Most insurers will still state, even on approved authorizations, that an authorization by itself does not guarantee payment, but they are still required when indicated by the insurer. If the insurer's handbook or policies document authorization requirements, then the only potential exceptions are granted for life-threatening emergency procedures that are evaluated on a case-by-case basis.

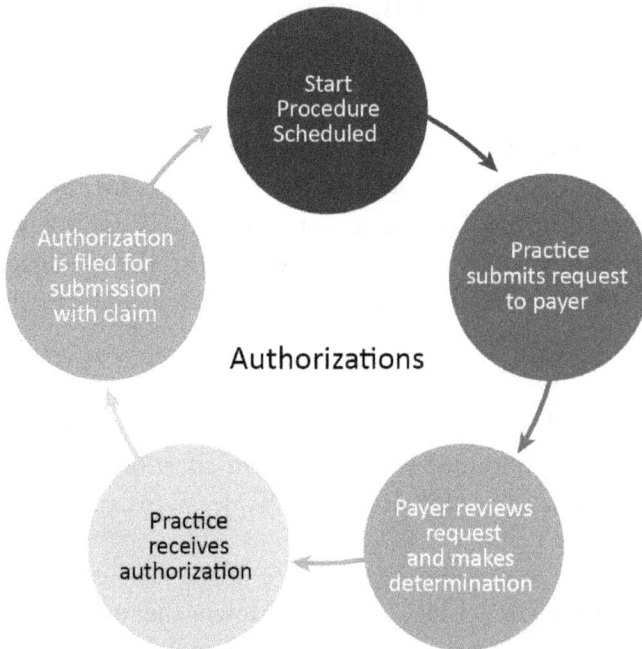

Figure 4.2   Authorization cycle

If the payer denies the procedure the practice can appeal or
provide documentation of additional therapies and resumbit.

Each insurance company will have their own process for requesting an authorization, but most insurance companies have an internet-based portal or method by which clinics can submit a form online that documents the procedure or medication requested. The form will generally require basic patient demographics, the patient's medical history (current diagnoses, previous diagnoses, symptoms, status, medications, etc.), and any other pertinent medical information.

For some insurance companies, this is still a paper form. This means a lot of handwritten papers, printing chart records and faxing things over to the insurance company. Regardless of the method, attention to detail is critical. Inaccurate information can result in denials, retracted payments and if done frequently, contract termination.

Retroactive authorizations are not approved often. There are still a few insurance companies that will do a retroactive authorization, but this is the exception, not the rule.

Without required authorizations, patients may be responsible for payment. The responsibility may also fall to the provider to contractually adjust off the balance based upon the provider's neglect to obtain the authorization.

Effective Authorization Plans

Developing an effective authorization process doesn't have to be difficult. There are easy steps that, once implemented, provide the checks and balances needed to have a successful program.

1. **A consistent identification method**

   Chances are that your practice already has a list of procedural codes from your fee schedule. (If not, see Chapter 11) Standard E&M codes like new patient visits and follow-up visits should not require authorization unless you do not participate with that payer. A billing specialist in your organization should create a quick reference guide for staff that schedule procedures and the staff that perform authorizations. Within the guide, the ability to reference by insurance company is most efficient, especially when combined with procedures which require authorization.

2. An authorization program and outlined steps

Authorization processes should be documented to give a reference to those who are new and to provide expectations for existing staff. Below are several key data elements that are needed when requesting prior authorization for medical services:

- Patient demographics
- Date of service and place of service
- Patient's insurance demographics
- Ordering provider name, NPI, provider number, and TIN
- Practice name, contact person, phone number, and fax number
- Diagnoses, service/procedure, CPT

3. Ongoing staff education

The employees who perform authorizations need to understand the role that the authorization plays in the billing process. They also need to understand the changes in payer regulations as they occur. The billing manager is responsible for following payer regulation changes, coverage updates, and authorization requirements. Information on the quick reference guides and any updates should be documented and verbally communicated to each prior-authorization employee.

4. Structured monitoring of authorization status

For those on electronic records, there is generally a way to enter a task or a "to-do" to follow-up on the status of the authorization. For those on paper charts, consider using a tickler system to keep track of the authorizations by status.

5. A proactive review period

Procedure schedulers should review all scheduled appointments for appropriate authorizations two or three business days before the procedures. Authorizations for any procedures that lack approval within 48-72 hours of procedure require updating. The employee should then follow pre-determined processes based upon the status.

6. **A documented plan for issue management**

   For example, if an employee identifies a missing authorization for a procedure scheduled in two business days, do they know what the next steps are? They should. Either obtain the authorization or reschedule the patient and fill the slot. Empty slots decrease projected revenue just as non-reimbursable procedures decrease projected revenue. Early identification alone will not resolve prior authorization issues, employees need to know the next steps to take. Key individuals should escalate issues and include critical information for inclusion.

7. **Documentation of final authorization determinations**

   Authorizations should be documented in the patient's chart whether approved or denied. For approvals, attach the authorization to outgoing claims. For denials, retain documentation to support redeterminations or as evidence to the patient.

8. **A process for benefits verification and coverage eligibility**

   Future services should have coverage verified to determine if a deductible or coinsurance would be applicable. Also, determine any out-of-pocket expenses the patient may have for the service.

For some insurance companies, the authorization is basic:

Approved 1/1/2019 - 1/31/2019 Laparoscopic Cholecystectomy 1.00 Unit(s)

Other insurance companies may send a separate document to the practice via payer portal, fax, or regular mail.

> COMPUTER Some EHRs are working on or have the capability to initiate pharmaceutical authorizations. As a provider community, we want to begin requesting that our EHR/PM software vendors provide assistance with requesting and tracking prior authorizations for services. In states that are working on standardizing the prior authorization process, including our software vendors in these efforts are important to close the loop on needs.

Case in Point: When Authorizations Don't Match the Procedure

Whenever possible, the authorization should match the procedure performed. Occasionally, the physician will need to change the procedure performed. This typically happens after the surgery has started and is usually due to patient safety concerns, unrealized severity, or additional complexities.

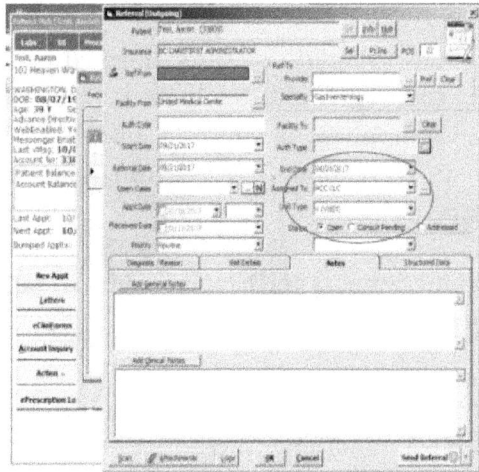

Figure 4.3   Example Referral Authorization screen

For example, if a provider goes in to perform a laparoscopic appendectomy and the appendix ruptures, the provider may need to perform an open surgery to safely and adequately resolve. The basic purpose of the procedure has not changed but the CPT® code has changed. In this situation, communicate the change in procedure code as soon as possible so that the staff can request a revised authorization from the insurer. If the reason is due to one of the three reasons listed above, the change will have a greater chance of approval.

Notably, there are other types of authorizations (for example, medication authorizations), but for the purposes of this text, we focused on procedural authorizations. Most EHRs and PMs provide a method to document authorizations so they link to appropriate claims.

Summary

Clean claims submissions may or may not require referrals and/or authorizations. Though these two processes are similar they cover different parts of the revenue cycle model. The negative impacts of missed authorizations and referrals can be avoided with communication, education, and consistency.

✏ Chapter 4 Knowledge Check

Eligibility, Referrals and Authorizations

Question #1:

A written document from a PCP to a specialist approving visits to the specialist is referred to as a _____.

Question #2:

Documented approval ahead of a procedure or medication is referred to as an _____.

Question #3:

Authorizations should be verified _____ prior to procedure.

Answers:
Q1: Referral
Q2: Authorization
Q3: 48-72 hours

Endnotes

1. Novitas Solutions: Advance Beneficiary Notice of Non-Coverage: https://www. novitas-solutions.com/webcenter/portal/MedicareJH/pagebyid?contentId=00108636

2. Novitas Solutions: Advance Beneficiary Notice of Non-Coverage: https://www. novitas-solutions.com/webcenter/portal/MedicareJH/pagebyid?contentId=00108636

Chapter 5

Appointment Confirmations

Performing appointment confirmations simply means contacting the patient to make sure they are aware of the day, time, provider's name, and location of their upcoming appointment. It also includes encouraging the patient to show up for that appointment at the time necessary to complete the check-in and clinical intake processes. Most practices already have a structured method for performing appointment confirmations. There is data supporting both manual methods and electronic methods, so practices should select the option that best fits their patient population, specialty and organization. The most critical piece of appointment confirmations is that they are performed consistently. Keep a steady process that staff may adhere to and patients can expect on a routine basis.

Methods

Manual appointment confirmations

The office staff, or a contracted third-party, contacts the patients directly via phone to confirm their upcoming appointment. This method takes more time and requires more effort but is touted by many as the most personal and effective approach. This method also affords the practice with the opportunity to speak with the patient directly and provide or obtain any additional information necessary prior to the date of service.

Electronic appointment confirmations

The scheduling system, usually the PM system generates automated reminder calls, texts, or emails that are sent to patients to confirm their upcoming appointment. This method is the fastest way to perform outreach to patients, especially when there is a high volume of individuals to contact. Some patients prefer the use of technology to obtain reminders but in contrast, this may be seen as a less personal approach that does not fit the brand of every practice.

The debate continues over which method is best, but, again, the key point here is that confirmations must be performed, regardless of your position on electronic or manual methods.

> COMPUTER Customize your EHR's appointment confirmation communication to give it a personal touch. Consider adding a picture of the patient's provider or of the office, include a link to an online map tool. You can also personalize the message patients receive via text and email. Determine the number and frequency of appointment reminders that are sent. It might be helpful to mindfully design the order the electronic appointments are sent (i.e., three reminders: first reminder by email two weeks prior to appointment, second reminder via text one week prior to appointment, third and final reminder 48 hours prior to appointment.)

Why Confirming Appointments Matters

The act of performing appointment confirmations has many benefits to the practice and patient such as:

1. Obtain updated patient information.

2. Remind patients of upcoming appointments.

3. Increase overall 'patient show' rates and decrease no show rates.

4. Address conditions before they exacerbate and require hospitalization.

5. Minimize emergency room visits by preventive care.

6. Foster a robust patient-provider relationship.

7. Make patients aware of old outstanding balances.

8. Provide patients with education on disease and medication management.

9. Managing provider and staff resource time by being aware of actual daily volumes.

10. Practice preparation of needed vaccines and other purchased visit materials.

Keeping the patient's information current is critical for billing purposes. For electronic methods, the method to verify patient information may require patient portal access. The confirmation process is a courtesy service to the patients that also provides a benefit to the organization. When patients need to cancel or reschedule, knowing ahead of time grants an opportunity to fill time slots. The confirmation contact, however it occurs, can be expected to drive improvement in patient attendance for appointments.

SHOUT OUT GUY   If you aren't sure, review the practice policy on leaving patient messages and look for that patient's privacy elections. To protect patient's privacy, consider the best approach for deciding how you identify yourself when leaving a message. If the practice specialty is included in the practice name, (i.e., XYZ Infectious Disease Specialists) consider excluding the practice name in your voice mail message and just leave the healthcare provider's last name (i.e., Dr. XYZ). If patients don't answer, leave a voicemail. Make sure to have a policy regarding patient voicemails and to obtain patient consent in advance. When leaving messages, be sure that the voicemail isn't being left in a general mailbox but rather is going directly to the patient.

Workflow

If the patient answers the phone during the appointment confirmation process, then the patient should follow one of two workflows:

Options A - Patient Confirms

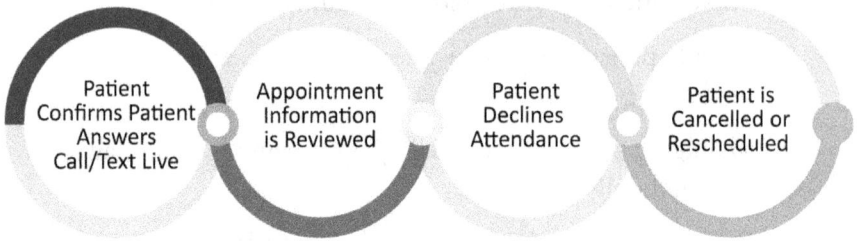

Figure 5.1   Option A – Patient Confirms

Options B - Patient Cancels/Reschedules

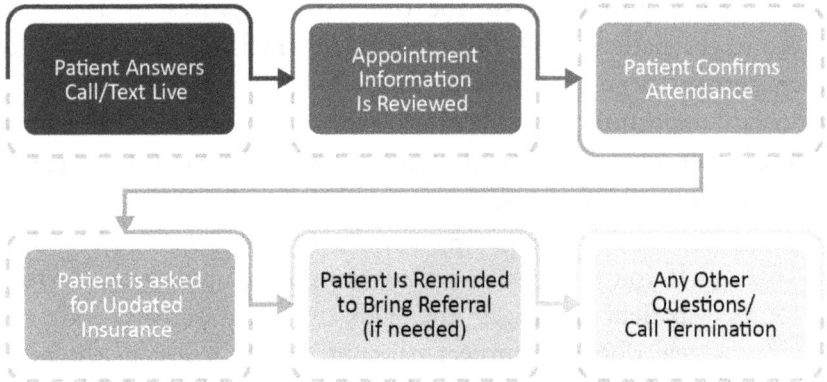

Figure 5.2   Option B – Patient Cancels or Reschedules

With Option B, the patient has canceled or rescheduled. There is now a hole in the schedule. There are different ways to fill this hole, i.e., selecting the next patient on the wait list, filling with other patients who call in for an appointment in the interim, etc. Educate the front desk on the importance of filling schedule holes. Prior to moving on, have staff attempt to reschedule patient's appointments while they are still on the phone.

Timing

You will want to perform appointment confirmations two business days prior to the date-of-service for a few reasons. Two days' notice allows time to fill schedule holes with new patients or wait-listed patients. During the confirmation call, some patients will realize they have a scheduling conflict and will cancel or move their appointment. Performing the confirmation call in advance allows staff to contact and schedule patients booked further out or patients who are on a waitlist.

It also allows time to identify and obtain missing referrals. Once identified, reach out to the patient's primary care office to obtain a referral for the upcoming appointment in advance. During this confirmation process, ask the patient about insurance changes and perform new benefit verifications.

Some patients will need to reschedule or cancel an appointment. Consider having a waiting list saved within your EHR for patients who are scheduled for appointments in the future but would be interested in being seen sooner and on short notice. These patients are viable candidates to fill schedule holes rather quickly.

Chart Preparation Process

This process is an investigation and review of key areas of the practice's transactions with or on behalf of a patient. It also allows the practice to identify and request needed information for a thorough office visit and enhanced patient experience. The chart prep process if conducted, should take place one to two days prior to the patient's appointment. It is a good idea to have the chart prep process coincide with the appointment confirmation process. Who wants to complete a comprehensive chart preparation for a patient who has cancelled their appointment during the confirmation process? The chart preparation process involves reviewing patient's records and accounts who have upcoming appointments for the following details.

Copays and Deductibles

If your practice utilizes paper superbills or electronic tasking, this is an excellent time to document the copay due at the TOS or the remaining patient deductible prior to a procedure. Collecting copays up front is critical to the revenue cycle model.

You can avoid wasting time and money chasing small patient balances by collecting these amounts due at the time of service. Train your staff in balance and copay identification and collection processes of each and make sure the chart preparation process involves some method of flagging the patient out of pocket expenses.

Outstanding Patient Balances

The billing department should document and flag outstanding patient balances in a way the front desk staff can recognize, and the front desk should be educated on the process for recognizing this information. Face-to-face appointments provide an excellent opportunity to collect overdue balances and setup payment plans. Have someone review patients' accounts to determine if they have been or are in danger of being sent to bad debt collections. It will be necessary to have a process in place for determining the appropriate course of action for patients who have outstanding balances but need to be seen.

Necessary Referrals

If a patient requires a referral for their upcoming visit and one is not on file, the chart prep process is the final check prior to the DOS. This gives the practice time to contact the patient or the patient's referring provider.

Referral forms may vary by insurance company or even by state. For example, the state of Maryland has a specific state form entitled the Maryland Uniform Consultation Referral form (MUCR).[1]

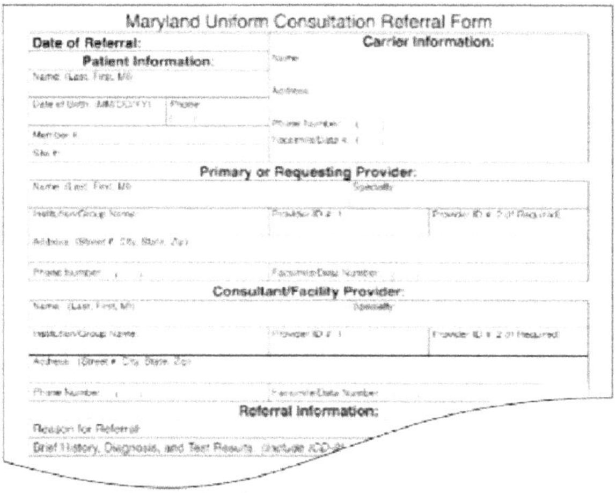

Maryland Uniform Consultation Referral Form

Date of Referral:

Patient Information:

Carrier Information:

Primary or Requesting Provider:

Consultant/Facility Provider:

Referral Information:

Figure 5.3 Maryland Uniform Consultation Referral form

Missing Labs or Imaging Requested

Most staff review the "Assessment & Plan" to get an idea of next steps in the provider's treatment plan in preparation for upcoming appointments. This is also a good time to ensure that all prior encounter notes are closed, locked and signed off by the provider.

Sometimes patients receive an order to get labs or imaging done prior to their next appointment. Staff should identify completion, providers review and filing of these reports in the patient's record during the chart preparation process. Develop a protocol for handling instances in which labs, imaging or external testing was ordered and not completed prior to the date of service. If the results of these tests were a requirement for the current visit, it might be best to consider rescheduling the patient if required labs or imaging have not been performed. Either way, resolve incomplete testing by making sure the patient still has the order for external testing, knows where to go to get the testing and that the results will be sent to your practice. Close the loop on incomplete testing to avoid additional delays in treatment.

Interpreter or Transportation Requirements

Unaddressed barriers to care may prevent patients from coming in for their appointments. Two common challenges are the need for interpreter services and the need for transportation. The chart prep process and appointment confirmation call may be the last opportunity for the office to help coordinate these external needs. ADA guidelines require that healthcare provider's offer, at the practice's expense, interpreting services.[2] Review these guidelines to ensure you are following all regulations. It may also be of benefit to check with your practice's accountant or tax preparer regarding potential write-offs for interpreting service expenses. Patients who are covered by an MCO will also have transportation resources. During the chart prep and/or appointment confirmation processes, be sure to discuss these needs with patient. Create patient account flags to alert staff of a patient's interpreter or transportation needs so an action plan may be developed prior to each office visit.

LIGHTBULB For quality reasons, make sure to review patient needs related to social determinants of health (SDOH). Build a method of review and a reference library of support services for staff to access when needed. If you are unfamiliar with SDOH, navigate to www.cdc.gov/ or to www.healthypeople.gov

SHOUT OUT GUY If your practice uses paper superbills, print them during the chart preparation process. Maintain all superbills regardless of patient attendance. Billing can mark balances due, referrals needed, and more, somewhere on the superbill accordingly: "no show," etc. This maintains consistency from billing to the front desk. Also consider utilizing a sign-in sheet to reconcile superbills at the end of day. For more information on superbills, navigate to the Chapter 9 section on superbills.

Chapter 5 Knowledge Check

Appointment Confirmations

Question #1:

This process can help identify that patients are missing a necessary referral:

Question #2:

The three main purposes of performing appointment confirmations are

_____

_____

_____

Question #3:

Chart prep occurs _____ day(s) before appointment.

Answers:

Q1: Chart Preparation

Q2: To update patient information, to remind patients about upcoming appointments, and to increase overall patient show rate.

Q3: 1-2

Endnotes

1. Maryland Uniform Consultation Referral Form (MUCR) https://mmcp.health. maryland.gov/epsdt/healthykids/AddendumSection5/Section-5-Addendum.pdf

2. ADA Effective Communication: https://www.ada.gov/effective-comm.htm

Chapter 6

Check-In & Time-of-Service Collections

Oh, the joys of check in and asking sick people for money! Who doesn't wake up in the morning and look forward to speaking the alien language of insurance guidelines and asking the elderly gentleman on a fixed income for his coinsurance payment? Although it can be a daunting task, one of the most critical components of the revenue cycle is the data collection process during check-in. Inaccurate data can result in lengthy claims denials and appeals processes. At check-in, some practices verify insurance, collect overdue balances, and update demographic data. According to *Becker's ASC Review*, "When the patient check-in process is not well-managed, physician practices not only experience decreased satisfaction, but also increased expense and lost revenue."[1]

A successful check-in process will include review of current patient demographics (see Appendix A for full list). Confirmation of patient demographics supports outreach to the patient's insurance carrier to verify the patient's coverage and payment responsibilities for the upcoming appointment.

If a patient has outstanding balances, collect them during check-in or prior to additional services being rendered. This includes amounts due for previously rendered services as well as copays or applicable deductible amounts. Whatever you do, avoid sending patient statements or invoices for copays; it's not financially feasible in most cases. See the end of Chapter 3 for some suggestions on approaches for addressing copays and deductibles.

Patient Contact Information and Demographics

It cannot be emphasized enough that patient demographic information needs to be regularly updated to ensure accuracy. This should start with the full name of the patient who is seeing the provider that day. If possible, confirm this information by requesting to see identification from the patient and match it with the insurance card and the demographic information you have on file for the patient. (See "Red Flag Rule" section in Chapter 16). When updating the patient's address, be sure to ask where the patient resides. As a point of clarification, also ask where the practice should send bills representing patient balances. Avoid accepting a post office box as the home address where a patient resides, as it becomes difficult to match insurance records to the patient for a post office box.

Provide a way to allow the patient to see the phone and email address the practice has on file and ask them to check for accuracy. One method is to print out a print screen of the demographics screen in the EHR/PM software and have the patient confirm all information. If there is a secure manner to do so, another option is to have the patient view an electronic version of their demographics in your system to validate information as being accurate. Whatever you do please, please, please don't ask the patient, "Has anything changed?" From the patient's perspective the answer could be misleading and result in inaccurate information. It is worthwhile finding out if their cell phone should be listed as primary phone number, as many individuals no longer have a landline at home. As mentioned earlier, be sure to have gained their consent to leave messages on an identified number's voicemail and

Confirm with the patient who is responsible for their bills or who the guarantor is. The insurance policy holder is not always the guarantor so confirming this person is important for the collections process. To be able to communicate with the guarantor regarding bills, obtain the phone, address, and email for the person who is the guarantor and/ or the insurance subscriber. If the policy is through the guarantor's employer, also obtain their employer's information and the guarantor's date of birth. This information is necessary for insurance verification and claims processing.

Finally, make sure to verify the insurance coverage information including the plan number, claims mailing address, member ID, and coordination of policies (primary, secondary, etc.).

COMPUTER   To enhance patients' in-office experience, consider allowing patients to have hands-on participation in the check-in and electronic form completion. There is also technology to take photos and accept eSignatures during the check-in process. Remember to set system parameters that allow your staff to stay involved in the check-in, while including the patient in the process.

To enhance patients' in-office experience, consider allowing patients to have hands-on participation in the check-in and electronic form completion. There is also technology to take photos and accept eSignatures during the check-in process. Remember to set system parameters that allow your staff to stay involved in the check-in, while including the patient in the process.

Assignment of Benefits and Consent to Treat

Many practices utilize a financial policy that outlines the practice's policies related to fees and patient's financial responsibility for medical and related services. The Assignment of Benefits (AOB) should be referenced in a financial policy.

Assignment of Benefits: AOB occurs when patients request that their insurance company send any and all payments applicable to the healthcare services provided sent directly to that provider.

The Assignment of Benefits (AOB) and the Consent to Treat are two critical documents for all healthcare entities. These forms, along with providing consent for treatment or admission, help to ensure that a provider obtains a right to payment from either the patient or the patient's health insurance. During the registration process, a patient will execute the AOB that allows the provider to seek reimbursement from the insurance company. Once treatment is provided, the care entity will submit the AOB and claim for payment. Upon process and approval of the claim, the insurance company will pay the provider directly. The goal is to avoid having to pursue payment from the patient unless there is a patient responsibility portion owed. The AOB's ultimate role is to create a more effective and efficient payment system.

While the execution of the AOB is crucial, more importantly, the healthcare provider needs to ensure that the language throughout the AOB is specific; vaguely written AOBs lead to fluid interpretations that may cause future claim contestations by payers. The healthcare entity's appeals rights and ability to file suit against the payer will depend on whether the provider has a valid and explicit AOB. Therefore, the entity needs to construct an AOB that will include specific language. AOBs should include language that directly speaks to "Assigning the Benefits and the Right to Sue and Receive Benefits." This language will protect the entity from payers, especially ERISA plans (employee insurance plans that cover healthcare services), that often seek to avoid payments to providers based on claims and AOBs. A substantial written AOB will drive payment efficacy and protect the provider entity's right to appeal and sue the insurance plan if the claim and/or AOB are disputed.

Charletta Washington, MHA – President, Precision Healthcare Solutions[2]

Insurance Verification

It is important to conduct benefits verifications, either through your software or directly through the payer. Many PM software's have built-in eligibility and benefits verification processes when a clearinghouse is directly interfaced. This is the preferred method of verification and documentation, because it's quick and it's time stamped. If that isn't an option for your practice, then verify both eligibility and benefit information via phone or through a payer's website portal.

The correct phone or website to use should be on the back of the patient ID card. Keep in mind this information is only useful if the insurance card is current. Therefore, make sure to obtain the patients current insurance card and to inquire as to whether they have received any new cards or made any changes to benefits recently.

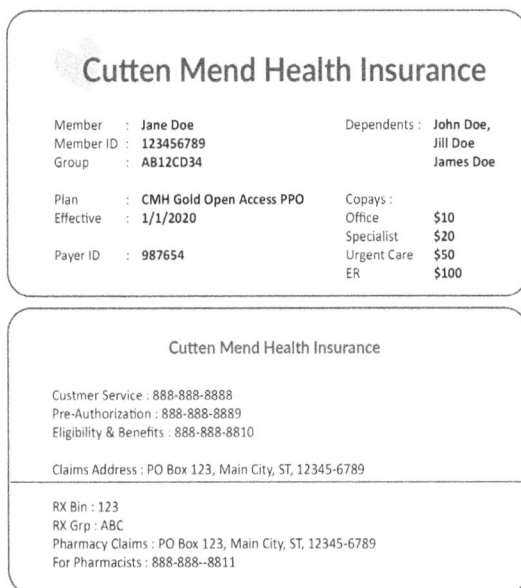

Figure 6.1   Front and Back of Example Health Insurance Card

Above is a sample patient ID card, all information
included is fictitious; this is for sample purposes only.

Regardless of the method (phone, portal, or EHR) the verification process should confirm or deny patient coverage, review outstanding deductibles, and give details on copayment / coinsurance amounts due by facility and specialty.

The practice will want to make sure to document the benefit verification information provided by insurance for each patient. For those performed electronically, documentation may be automatic. For phone verifications, a carefully defined process will aid in proper and complete documentation. This becomes significant during the claim's adjudication process. Proof of eligibility verification supports the appeals process for coverage-based claims denials. See the Appendix I for competency standards for staff who are conducting benefits verifications.

Different Types of Insurance

As we leverage the information received during the check-in process for billing, we also need to understand the historical context of each financial class to understand and follow their reimbursement guidelines.

Federal

Medicare

This is the most widely known federal insurance program. Medicare-eligible beneficiaries are usually those age 65 or older, or eligible beneficiaries under the age of 65 if they have qualifying disabilities. Medicare eligibility does require historical contribution into the Medicare program. Contribution to the Medicare program prior to eligibility usually occurs in the form of pre-tax payroll deductions. More information on eligibility, is available at www.medicare.gov.

In accordance with federal policy, Medicare outlines all reimbursement schedules and program requirements at www.cms.gov. The Medicare rates are so widely known and easily accessed that practice charge masters often use the Medicare Physician Fee Schedule (PFS) as a benchmark against other payer reimbursement schedules. For more on charge masters, navigate to Chapter 11 – Payment Posting.

To improve security and protect patient's identities, Medicare began issuing new versions of insurance cards. For instance, Social Security numbers have been removed from the insurance cards. The new cards were mailed to patients between April 2018 and April 2019. There are significant differences in the new Medicare insurance cards, including new unique Medicare numbers. For more information for providers and office managers, refer to https://www.cms.gov/Medicare/New-Medicare-Card/Providers/Providers-and-office-managers.html. Patients should be referred to https://www.medicare.gov/forms-help-resources/your-medicare-card.

Medicare Administrative Contractor (MAC)

According to CMS:

> *A Medicare Administrative Contractor (MAC) is a private healthcare insurer that has been awarded a geographic jurisdiction to process Medicare Part A and Part B (A/B) medical claims or Durable Medical Equipment (DME) claims for Medicare Fee-For-Service (FFS) beneficiaries. CMS relies on a network of MACs to serve as the primary operational contact between the Medicare FFS program and the healthcare providers enrolled in the program. MACs are multi-state, regional contractors responsible for administering both Medicare Part A and Medicare Part B claims. MACs perform many activities including:*

> - *Process Medicare FFS claims*
> - *Make and account for Medicare FFS payments*
> - *Enroll providers in the Medicare FFS program*
> - *Handle provider reimbursement services and audit institutional provider cost reports*
> - *Handle redetermination requests (1st stage appeals process)*
> - *Respond to provider inquiries*

- *Educate providers about Medicare FFS billing requirements*
- *Establish local coverage determinations (LCDs)*
- *Review medical records for selected claims*
- *Coordinate with CMS and other FFS contractors*[3]

Redeterminations: An independent review of an initial determination. A redetermination is conducted by the same Medicare contractor that issued the initial determination and refers to the decision made in the first level of the Medicare appeals process.

Some states have only one MAC, while others have several. For example, Texas has eight MAC localities. Each MAC locality has a different geographic adjustment factor (GAF) applied and reimbursement guidelines may vary as well. When using the CMS Physician Fee Schedule Lookup tool[4] or your MAC website, refer to your MAC locality for accurate rates. Refer to the CMS website and use your practice address to confirm your MAC and MAC locality.

Tricare

Tricare is a coverage program for active duty and retired members of the US military and their families. Tricare has a variety of plans, including Prime (which is an HMO), Select, For Life, and West, among others. Benefits may include military spouses, dependents, and National Guard members as well. Tricare may act as a secondary insurance and may cover deductible amounts of the primary payer. The circumstances for coverage vary. For more information, navigate to https://health.mil and search for "Tricare."

State/Medicaid

Medicaid coverage is funded and regulated at both the federal and state level. This can lead to confusion regarding rules as there may be conflicting policies. In general, the strictest rule applies, but when in doubt, contact the state office for Medicaid. Some states offer "straight Medicaid" only, meaning the plan management is through the state

Medicaid office. Other states offer MCOs. That Medicaid.gov defines as "a healthcare delivery system organized to manage cost, utilization, and quality."[5] Most states offer both Medicaid MCOs and straight Medicaid; navigating to your state Medicaid website is a great way to review plan requirements and payment policies. If a patient selects a Medicaid MCO, claims must be billed to that specific MCO instead of being sent directly to Medicaid. Patients who have selected a Medicaid MCO will also be able to switch to a different MCO, so it is necessary to verify benefits prior to each office visit.

Commercial

There are four well-known "giants" in commercial insurance: Aetna, Anthem, Cigna, and UnitedHealthcare. Humana and Kaiser also have large national consumer bases. Each of these insurers have an array of health plans, including HMO plans, PPO plans, Medicare Advantage plans, etc. The type of health plan a patient is covered with will help determine the patient's out-of-pocket expectations. Unfortunately, most patients do not understand these differences or how the variances impact cost and coverage. Having staff who serve as educators or "Patient Financial Services" will assist patients with understanding their coverage. The most common are below with key differentiators:

Table 6. 1 Insurance Card Identification Guidance

	HMO	PPO	EPO	POS	HDHP
Premium	Low	Higher	Variable	Variable	Low
Deductible	Low	Variable	Variable	Variable	Very High
PCP	Must be set	Typically open	Typically open	May be set	Typically open
Copays	Normal or non-existent	Normal to high	Normal to high	Normal to high	Generally paid through HSA
In-Network	Average width	Fairly open	Less open than PPO	Very broad	Average
Referral to Specialists?	Usually	No	No	Usually	No
Out-of-Network Coverage	Minimal to none	Variable	Minimal to none	Some	Minimal to none

Specialist: Healthcare provider who focuses on a certain medical discipline. This provider focuses on managing, diagnosing, and treating certain illnesses and symptoms. There is usually specialized training or board certification for the specialized area of medicine.

Neighboring states may have insurance companies in common. Some insurance plans will cross state lines; this is an important factor when you're selecting the payer for patient registration, so that payer adjudication occurs through the correct claims processing center. This is also an important factor during the credentialing process to ensure you are requesting participation with the appropriate insurance plans based on your practice location and the corresponding regions for the payer. In both cases, you need to be aware of regulations that may differ from state-to-state. Review MAC Localities and commercial payer coverage maps for greater understanding. For example, the Maryland, DC, Virginia area has examples of cross-state commercial plans and Medicare localities: may differ from state-to-state. Review MAC Localities and commercial payer coverage maps for greater understanding. For example, the Maryland, DC, Virginia (DMV) area has examples of cross-state commercial plans and Medicare localities:

- Per CMS, MAC Locality# 1220201 covers Washington, D.C. and certain suburbs of Maryland and Virginia which are in close proximity.
- Carefirst BCBS has plans that span Maryland, DC, and Northern Virginia while their counterpart, Anthem, services the remainder of Virginia.

Liability

These coverage plans come into effect when accidents occur. Workers compensation policies, motor vehicle accidents, personal injury protection (PIP) etc. A case manager, who is responsible for defining allowable visits, approving referrals, and authorizing payment for services, often fully manages these policies. There might be a claim associated to the injury that will need to be included in billing submissions and prior authorizations as needed.

Contact case managers before rendering services for liability policies. Emergency services are the only exception to this rule. For any new problem discussed, ask patients if the problem is related to a work or vehicle accident. In the event a medical problem is unrelated to an injury claim, that service is likely going to be denied. It's important to separate and differentiate care being given for an injury as opposed to non-injury related services when billing liability insurance. It is equally as important to select the appropriate corresponding diagnosis code for injury-related services to avoid claim adjudication confusion. On the flip side, selecting an injury code as a primary diagnosis may be denied by a health insurance plan as they may expect liability coverage to pay for the injury claims.

Coordination of Benefits

It is common for patients to have more than one type of insurance. For example, they may have Medicare and Medicaid, or may have Medicare as well as coverage through a spouse's employer. In situations in which patients have more than one insurance, there is a specific billing order or sequence for each insurance policy. The order of billing is known as the coordination of benefits (COB).

The primary payer, as the name suggests, pays first. Send any remaining amount (coinsurance, deductible, etc.) to the secondary payer. The secondary payer will pay next, and, if the patient has three coverage policies, the claim will then need to go to the tertiary payer.

If you suspect that a patient may have more than one type of insurance coverage, take the time to research and obtain all pertinent information to ensure practice records are accurate. Correct data entry during registration is key to accurately billing insurances in the proper order.

Most practices no longer submit paper claims or have the hassle of printing secondary claims. Medicare will automatically cross-file claims to the secondary insurance payer

Many clearinghouses, practice management systems, and third-party billers will also automatically submit to the secondary insurance payer. In the event you notice that your secondary claims are not being paid, check to see if there is an issue with Electronic Data Interchange (EDI) numbers or the clearinghouse interface for cross-filing.

> **Cross-file:** This is the process by which claims are submitted electronically to the next payer responsible. For example, a primary payer sending a copy of their EOB to the secondary payer on file.

Medicare

If a patient has Medicare coverage, then Medicare will typically pay first, but there are exceptions to this. For example, if a Medicare patient also has group coverage under their spouse's employer group health plan (EGHP), then Medicare bills secondary to the EGHP, if the EGHP is for more than twenty employees. Understanding COB for Medicare can be challenging. For more information navigate to www.medicare.gov and enter the search term "coordination of benefits." It is recommended that you utilize a Medicare Secondary Payer (MSP) questionnaire process to determine Medicare's sequencing in the coordination of benefits process.

For additional details on Medicare Coordination of Benefits and MSP, navigate to: https://www.cms.gov/Medicare/Coordination-of-Benefits-and-Recovery/ Coordination-of-Benefits-and-Recovery-Overview/Medicare-Secondary-Payer/Downloads/ MSP-Overview.pdf

Medicaid

Medicaid almost always pays last and there are very few exceptions to this rule, which is why many refer to Medicaid as the *payer of last resort*. Once Medicaid has paid their allowable amount, it is unlawful to bill the patient for any additional premium. The only exception to this would be amounts which Medicaid deems the patient responsibility. Adjust non-allowed amounts as dictated on the EOB. There are some Medicaid MCOs that include a small coinsurance or copayment amount from their patients.

Working Aged & Employer Group Health Plan (GHP)	Beneficiary is 65 or older, currently employed and covered by a GHP or covered by a spouse's GHP AND employer has LESS than 20 employees. [MEDICARE PAYS PRIMARY] Beneficiary is 65 or older, currently employed and covered by a GHP or covered by a spouse's GHP AND employer has MORE than 20 employees. [MEDICARE PAYS SECONDARY TO GHP INSURANCE] Beneficiary is 65 or older, self-employed and covered by a GHP or covered by spouse's GHP AND employer has MORE than 20 employees. [MEDICARE PAYS SECONDARY TO GHP INSURANCE]
Disability & Employer GHP	Beneficiary is disabled, covered by their employers current GHP or through a family member's GHP AND the employer has 100 or MORE employees. [MEDICARE PAYS SECONDARY TO GHP INSURANCE]
ESRD	Beneficiary has End Stage Renal Disease (ESRD), is in the first 30 months of Medicare entitlement, and is covered by a GHP. [MEDICARE PAYS SECONDARY DURING 30-MONTH COB PERIOD FOR ESRD] Beneficiary has End Stage Renal Disease (ESRD), is in the first 30 months of Medicare entitlement, and is covered by a COBRA Plan. [MEDICARE PAYS SECONDARY DURING 30-MONTH COB PERIOD FOR ESRD]
COBRA	Beneficiary is covered by COBRA and is in the first 30 months of Medicare entitlement. [MEDICARE PAYS SECONDARY DURING 30-MONTH COB PERIOD FOR ESRD] Beneficiary is 65 or older and has Medicare & COBRA. [MEDICARE PAYS SECONDARY TO COBRA] Beneficiary is disabled and covered by Medicare & COBRA. [MEDICARE PAYS PRIMARY]
Retiree Health	Beneficiary is 65 or older and has a an employer retirement plan. [MEDICARE PAYS PRIMARY TO RETIREE COVERAGE]
No-fault Insurance	Beneficiary is eligible for Medicare and was involved in an accident where liability or no-fault insurance is paying for services. [MEDICAREPAYS SECONDARY TO LIABILITY/NO FAULT INSURANCE]
Worker's Comp	Benficiary is eligible for Medicare and has Worker's Compensation coverage due to a job-related injury or illness. [MEDICARE USUALLY WILL NOT PAY FOR CLAIMS RELATED TO WORKER'S COMP.]

Figure 6.2   Determining Medicare's Primary or Secondary Responsibility

Dual-Eligible Beneficiaries

This term identifies patients who have both Medicare and Medicaid. For these patients, claims are "paid in full" if both Medicare and Medicaid have paid. It is prohibited to seek additional reimbursement from a patient once Medicare and Medicaid have paid. For more information on dual eligible billing, navigate to www.cms.gov and enter the search term "dual eligible beneficiaries".

Liability

When liability policies apply, bill all DOS related to the patient's liability claim to the liability policy. Coordination of benefits thereafter are case by case. If a claim number is required, be sure that it is accurately listed on the claim form for submission. If possible, attempt to obtain the claim adjuster's name and contact information for assistance with claims payment.

SHOUT OUT GUY   If your practice utilizes a third-party biller, make sure to review the conditions and process for submission of claims to other payers. Most federal and commercial insurers will deny claims related to a no-fault, PIP, Workers Compensation, or illness/injury case. For example, some third-party billing companies will not submit tertiary claims. It is critical to understand the boundaries of your third-party billing company and to audit their activity for accuracy and compliance.

If your practice utilizes a third-party biller, make sure to review the conditions and process for submission of claims to other payers. Most federal and commercial insurers will deny claims related to a no-fault, PIP, Workers Compensation, or illness/injury case.

For example, some third-party billing companies will not submit tertiary claims. It is critical to understand the boundaries of your third-party billing company and to audit their activity for accuracy and compliance.

Insurance Database Management

PM systems provide a method for storing insurance plans. Utilize that methodology to create a database for easy plan retrieval when entering patient insurance demographic information.

Usually the database will allow you to create groupings and codes to help you organize the database. Consider grouping insurance first by type (federal, Medicaid, liability, etc.) and then by payer. There will be multiple plans for each payer, so grouping them and thinking about your code methodology helps save time for your team. For information on grouping payers by financial class, go to Chapter 15.

For example, if all your Medicare Advantage Plans begin with MA, your staff can easily navigate to the right plan section when entering new patient insurance information. Examples below:

MA001 – Cutten Mend Medicare Advantage Plan
MA002 – Humanoid Medicare Advantage Plan
MA003 – Green Tea Medicare Advantage Plan

> **Medicare Advantage Plan:** Health benefits coverage offered under a policy or contract by a Medicare Advantage organization that includes a specific set of health benefits offered at a uniform premium and uniform level of cost-sharing to all Medicare beneficiaries residing in the service area of the Medicare Advantage plan.

The accuracy of this database is critical to efficient claims processing. If your staff selects the wrong plans during registration, this can result in claims denials, and overall RCM challenges. Consider creating a reference guide for your front desk to support their decision making when selecting insurance payers

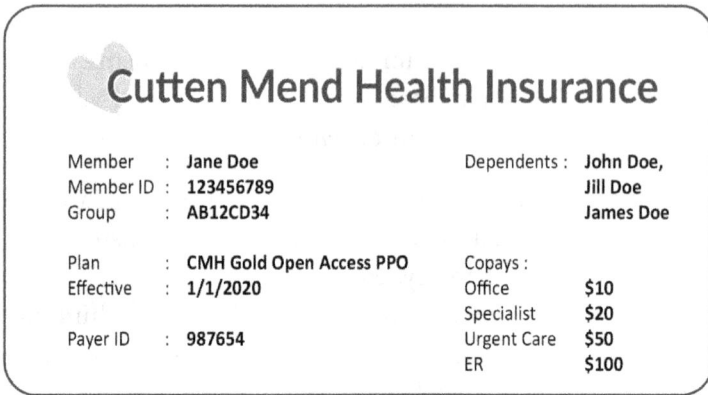

Figure 6.3   Example insurance card face

For example, if the patient presents a card like the one shown here (Figure 6.3), the reference guide may appear as Table 6.1 above. The table above refers the patient to verify specific information to confirm the right plan.

Providing a current and detailed reference guide alongside an accurate and well-maintained database will prevent unnecessary revenue cycle delays. If possible, consider removing insurance payers from your database that you do not participate with or payer selections in which the claims address is outdated or incorrect.

Insurance Contract Language

Each insurance company has provider participation guidelines that are spelled out in each unique participation agreement. This language explains the payer and the provider's obligations and expectations for participation, payment and care. The contract language within an insurance participation agreement is important to understand prior to agreeing upon it. Each insurance contract is unique and there are key terms and conditions to be aware of within each contract.

Timely Filing & Appeals Limits	Term (Effective & Expiration Date)	Termination (with or without cause)	Automatic Renewals
Correspondence Address	Contract Addendums	Malpractice coverage limits	Fee Schedule
Group or Individual contract	Utilization Management / Pre-Auth	Quality Management	Medical Necessity
Hold Harmless	Interest for Late Payments	Imposition of fee reductions	Adjustments / Recoupments

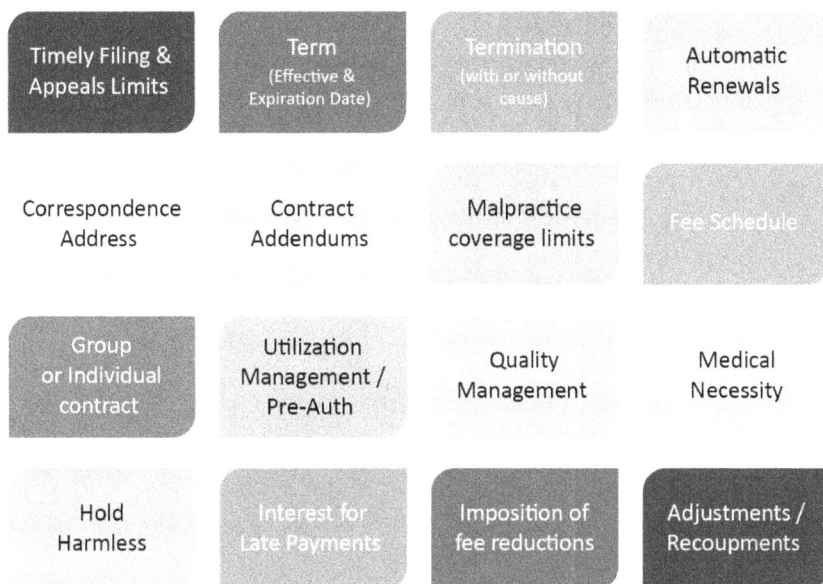

Figure 6.4   Key Terms and Conditions in Insurance Contracts

Required Collections

Most payer/provider contracts prohibit writing off patient copay, deductible and coinsurance without a qualified exception (such as a verified financial hardship). The practice is allowed to assess patients for exception on a case-by case basis, but you should have a set process to determine when exceptions can be made and fairly apply the process to all patients.

OIG's Opinion on Routine Copay Waivers

In 1994, the OIG released a special comment on the routine waiver of copays and remarked that, "routine waiver of deductibles and copayments by charge-based providers, practitioners, or suppliers is unlawful because it results in (1) false claims, (2) violations of the anti-kickback statute, and (3) excessive utilization of items and services paid for by Medicare." They further remarked that

> . . . a provider, practitioner or supplier who routinely
> waives Medicare copayments or deductibles is

misstating its actual charge. For example, if a supplier claims that its charge for a piece of equipment is $100, but routinely waives the copayment, the actual charge is $80. Medicare should be paying 80% of $80 (or $64), rather than 80%t of $100 (or $80). As a result of the supplier's misrepresentation, the Medicare program is paying $16 more than it should for this item. [9]

False Claims Act: This Act states that anyone who has knowingly submitted false claims to the government is liable to be penalized. The statute provides that one who is liable must pay a civil penalty and treble the amount of the government's damages.

Balance Billing

Balance Billing: Occurs when a healthcare provider charges/bills a patient for balance between the provider's charge amount which was billed to insurance and the allowed amount; which, for participating providers is the contract rate. Participating providers are not permitted to balance bill patients.

Once a claim is paid, an out-of-network physician, not contracted with a payer to accept in-network rate agreements, can bill patients for the entire remaining balance; this practice is known as balance billing. For example, if an out-of-network provider charges $150 for a service as usual, customary, and reasonable (UCR), but the insurance company only allowed $120, the provider may choose to bill the remaining balance of $30. The practice of balance billing is growing, according to Becker's Hospital Review, "Balance billing is on the rise nationally. In 2011, around 8% of privately insured individuals used out-of-network care, 40% of which resulted in unanticipated medical costs due to balance billing."[11] Balance billing is a derivative of battles between healthcare organizations and insurance carriers over fair reimbursement for medical providers. The practice of balance billing can find patients caught in the middle and facing unforeseen healthcare bills with potential negative financial impact on the patient.

Balance billing is a legal process if the provider is not contracted with the insurance company. Balance billing is an illegal act if a bill is sent to a client even though the provider is contracted with the client's insurance company. It is important to know the difference when you are executing contracts in your practice.[10]

Charletta Washington, MHA – President, Precision Healthcare Solutions

Usual, Customary, and Reasonable (UCR): The amount a health plan pays for covered medical services based on factors including geography and based on the charge amount providers charge for that or similar healthcare services.

Active/Inactive Rule

Insurance through the patient's employer will most likely be listed as the primary insurance. Insurance plans that the patient continues to be covered by after the patient is retired or laid off would be the secondary insurance after any insurance provided by an active employment.

Birthday Rule

For pediatric care, the birthday rule is a method of determining which parent's medical coverage will be primary for dependent children. The primary coverage will be the parent whose birth month and day falls first in the calendar year. If both parents have the same birthday, then the parent whose insurance plan has been effective for the longest period would be the primary for dependent children.

Non-Dependent/Dependent Rule

When sequencing the order of a patient's benefits, the plan that covers the patient as an employee or subscriber will be the primary insurance. The plan that the patient is listed as a dependent of another individual should be listed as secondary.

Patient Payments

Repeat patients may have outstanding account balances when they come into the office. Check-in is an excellent time to capture a payment. This is often referred to as TOS collections, which simply means the collection of copays, prospective payments, and outstanding balances on the date services are rendered.

Capturing payments from patients can be challenging, especially once they leave the facility. The front desk should attempt to capture outstanding payments at all face-to-face patient opportunities.

Financial Hardship

At any time, patients may disclose financial hardships, make sure you are aware of the financial hardship program at your practice. It is not acceptable to engage in blanket write-off of copays and other patient responsibilities. However, when patients truly have a financial hardship and meet the program requirements of the organization, then payment plans or write-offs may be appropriate.

A sample financial hardship application has been included in the appendices of this book. See Appendix G for more information. Feel free to customize this resource to fit the needs of your organization and have a set policy by which these applicants are approved or denied financial hardship waivers.

The OIG has commented on financial hardship waivers in many cases; refer to these special comments for additional guidance.[12]

Payment Plans

Patients with significant medical expenses or high-deductible health plans may find themselves with large balances they are unable to pay in full. Be sure to have a policy for the front desk on next steps and educate staff on properly implementing that policy. This policy should be reviewed annually to see if amendments are needed. If patients decline to make payment in full during check-in, the front desk must know how to proceed. Some options include having a financial counselor on hand, setting payment plans for the patient to choose from, and facilitating a mandatory conversation with management.

As patients' out-of-pocket expenses continue to increase with high-deductible plans and other cost-sharing models, healthcare providers must provide payment flexibility to their patients while adjusting their perspective on how they once viewed the patient-provider relationship. Patients have a choice in the provider they select and now can score providers in a variety of ways. With this knowledge, providers must consider patients as *buyers* of healthcare services they are *selling*. The provider as *seller* must conform to their *buyers* various financial needs to strengthen the buyer-seller relationship.

Payment Types

Cash and Check

Though cash and check payments seem to be waning, there is still a large population of patients that pay with these methods. Cash and check collections at the front desk can be challenging to reconcile and create an opportunity for company theft. To review appropriate internal controls for cash and check deposits, refer to Chapter 10.

SHOUT OUT GUY

Security Reminder: If using an online portal, make sure that each employee has their own login and password. This supports PCI compliance.

Credit Cards

Implementing a merchant services terminal is very common for payment of healthcare services. There are separate terminal machines that can work plug-and-play with an open phone line, or alternatively a plug-and-play computer USB that transacts through an online portal. Accepting credit cards is necessary, as we do not want to implement obstacles for payment. You will want to keep an eye on transaction fees and details such as when using a patient portal, your merchant services vendor may require higher online credit card transaction fees.

You should educate the individuals working at the front desk in the appropriate use of the credit card transaction equipment.

SHOUT OUT GUY **Policy Don't:** Do not allow employees to keep credit cards on file in unsecured locations with or without the patient's consent.

Payment Posting

Some practices post patient payments immediately upon receipt at the front desk; others send the payments back to the billing department for processing. There are ways to securely structure each program. Having a set policy on preferred process for different payment posting scenarios will help ensure smooth RCM.

Additionally, having payments posted at TOS will help reduce the opportunity for theft and is recommended where possible. For more information, refer to Chapter 11.

Check Out

Now that the visit is complete, the patient is ready to leave the office. Patients will view checkout delays as an inconvenience, but before we conclude the visit, we want to be sure that they have everything they need from us and that we have everything we need from them. Many practices utilize the same staff who may have checked the patient in to also check them out. If that's not the case, it's ideal to make sure patients know where to go to conclude their visit.

To ensure patients go through the check-out process, it's important to have a sign navigating patients to the appropriate check out location. When patients skip check out, we miss out on opportunities to not only provide patients with a summary of their visit but to also do the following:

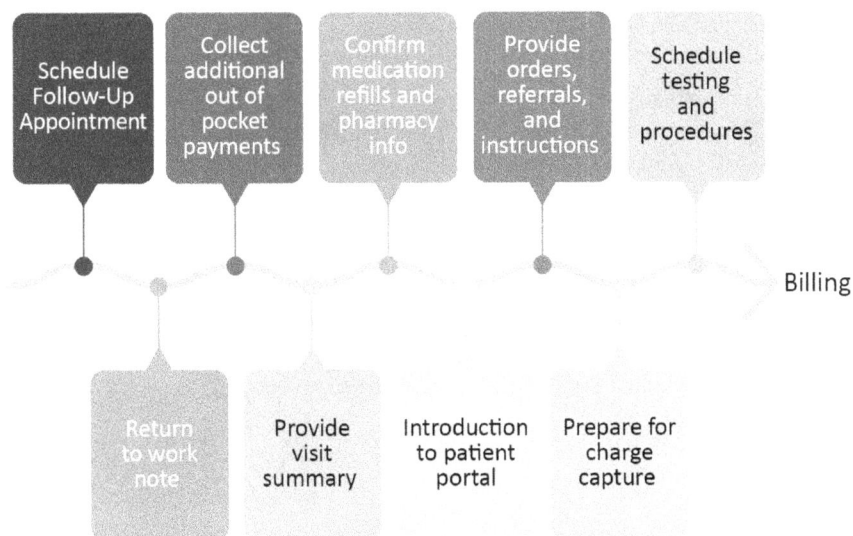

Figure 6.6   Check-out process

Reduced office phone calls are an important operational component seen in each of the above. The check-out process reduces the amount of incoming phone calls to the practice, and an effective check-out process can streamline workflows while improving customer service.

This is our last opportunity to address any patient concerns prior to their departure from the office. As our staff have knowledge of each patient's visit, they will be equipped to manage an effective check-out process.

For example, let's say our check-out staff is aware that a patient was seen for a pre-operative clearance. While patients are still onsite, they may need surgical instructions, prior-authorization, knowledge of coinsurance, and they may need to schedule a post-surgical follow-up appointment. It is important to complete as much as possible prior to the patient leaving the office so the patient is all set for surgery. If the employees performing check-out do not understand the visit process or standard protocols, then the check-out process may not be as effective as possible. Provide education to the front desk staff so they have a baseline understanding of visit types. For example, patients coming in for a pre-operative assessment should already have a prior authorization in place for the upcoming surgery. In this case, the visit type signals a need to verify a required document and proper education provides a critical check and balance to the revenue cycle.

Coinsurance: The remaining balance for a covered service that is the patient's responsibility to pay. Coinsurance is a percent of the allowed amount for a covered service. A calculation example is: Insurance pays 80% and leaves 20% as a coinsurance/patient responsibility. Many high-deductible health policies include a patient coinsurance.

We've already established the best practice of collection of money during TOS at check-in. However, there are instances in which payments must be collected after service is provided. In the event the patient has a coinsurance and the CPT code will not be determined until after the service, the patient's balance may not be collected until after the provider has determined the service level. When collecting coinsurances, there are several factors to consider:

Collecting coinsurance at the TOS is tricky. Unless you have real-time adjudication data, it may be difficult to accurately determine what claims have already been applied to a patient's deductible. Some practices prefer to allow the claim to be adjudicated and bill the patient; others perform these calculations at check out and collect prior to the patient exiting.

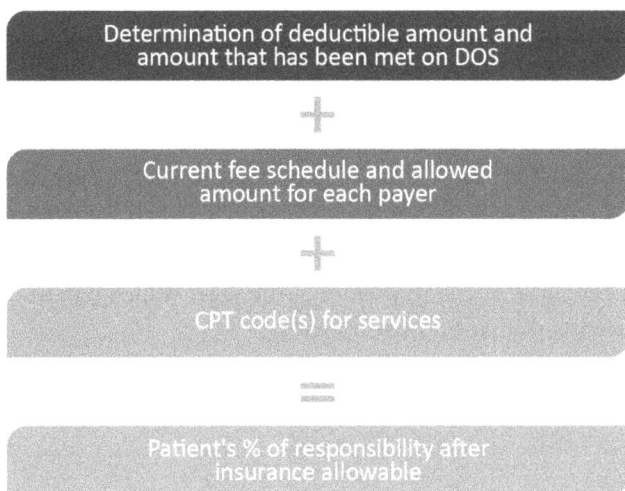

Figure 6.7   Factors to consider when collecting coinsurances

Customer Service

With so many key tasks to perform, it can be easy to go about check in and check out in a mechanical matter, but it's important to remember that your front desk is the greatest point of customer service that your patients will remember. You will find the investment in a staff well-trained in customer service is well worth it. When hiring for those pivotal front-desk positions, you will want to prioritize people who have a warm and welcoming demeanor. As the first face patients see when they arrive, and the last face they see when leaving, these employees create a lasting impression. In fact, some practices have begun renaming front desk positions to things like "Director of First Impressions."

Customer service is much more than just a warm smile, though. It means following-up with those patients who've had a long wait, keeping them informed of appointment delays, and ensuring patients' non-medical questions have been answered. Consider providing structured training to your front desk staff to ensure their knowledge of customer services best practices. MGMA provides excellent resources in print and online education to support these efforts.

✏ Chapter 6 Knowledge Check

Check-in and Time of Service Collections

Question #1:

A child shows up for pediatric care escorted by her grandmother. The grandmother has copies of both the mother and father's insurance cards. The parents have the same birthday, including the year. Which parent's insurance should be listed as primary responsibility?

Question #2:

Medicare and Tricare are two examples of _____ payers.

Question #3:

True or False? Routine copay waivers are essential and appropriate.

Question #4:

The amount a health plan pays for covered medical services based on factors including geography and based on the amount providers charge for that or similar healthcare services is the _____ amount.

Question #5:

True or False? Medicare Administrative Contractors (MACs) vary by state and some states may have more than one.

Question #6:

Why should you avoid accepting post office box addresses from patients?

Answers:

Q1: The parent whose insurance plan has been effective for the longest
Q2: Federal
Q3: False
Q4: Usual, Customary, and Reasonable (UCR)
Q5: True
Q6: It becomes difficult to match insurance records to the patient.

Endnotes

1. Diagnosing your patient check-in process: 4 ways to improve value. *Written by Eric Anderson, COO, Clearwave Corporation* | April 12, 2017 | https://www.beckersasc.com/or-clinical-quality/diagnosing-your-patient-check-in-process-4-ways-to-improve-value.html

2. Book quote provided by: *Charletta Washington, MHA – President, Precision Healthcare Solutions*

3. CMS: "What Is a MAC?" https://www.cms.gov/Medicare/Medicare-Contracting/Medicare-Administrative-Contractors/What-is-a-MAC.html

4. CMS Physician Fee Schedule Lookup Tool https://www.cms.gov/Medicare/Medicare-Fee-for-Service-Payment/PFSlookup/index.html

5. Medicaid.gov: Managed Care https://www.medicaid.gov/medicaid/managed-care/index.html

6. https://www.cms.gov/Regulations-and-Guidance/Guidance/Manuals/Downloads/clm104c23.pdf

7. CMS: "COB Fact Sheets: MSP Laws and Third Party Payers Fact Sheet for Attorneys" https://www.cms.gov/Medicare/Coordination-of-Benefits-and-Recovery/EmployerServices/Downloads/MSP-Laws-and-Third-Party-Payers-Fact-Sheet-for-Attorneys.pdf

8. CMS: "Medicare Secondary Payer"

9. OIG Special Fraud Alert, 12/19/1994 https://oig.hhs.gov/fraud/docs/alertsandbulletins/121994.html

10. Book Quote provided by: *Charletta Washington, MHA – President, Precision Healthcare Solutions*

11. 20 things to know about balance billing: As payers and https://www.beckershospitalreview.com/finance/20-things-to-know-about-balance-billing.html

12. OIG https://oig.hhs.gov/fraud/docs/alertsandbulletins/121994.html

Chapter 7

Documentation & Coding Background

It's safe to say that not all medical practice staff and providers are coding experts or even employ coding experts such as certified coders. However, understanding coding and documentation principles are essential skills for staff and providers to be able to provide excellent patient care, remain compliant, and have a successful revenue cycle.

Medical assistants and nursing staff need to have a baseline understanding of documentation and coding as they are assisting providers with gathering and documenting information such as chief complaint, medical history, medications and vital signs. Front office staff in some instances are triaging incoming calls and using this information to schedule medical office visits that initiate the documentation process. Billing staff use documentation and coding information in claim submission, denial prevention, and denial management. Providers are penultimately responsible for documenting a medical record and coding illnesses and services; however, many providers lack training in these areas. Practice leaders must oversee all roles related to documentation and coding, while mitigating practice risk, ensuring compliance, as well as ensuring maximum appropriate reimbursement.

The information contained within the medical record is extracted and converted into codes. These codes are used to articulate and justify the services rendered: illnesses, conditions, injuries, medications, and supplies, all of which have financial implications.

It cannot be emphasized enough that accurate and complete medical record documentation is a key piece of the revenue cycle. An accurate depiction of a patient's health record allows for optimal patient care as well as optimal reimbursement.

Medical Record Documentation

The primary purpose of clinical documentation is to tell the story of the medical care rendered. When medical records are not completed accurately, it can result in payment denials, audit recoupments, and other financial impacts related to errors in care delivery. This means the process of *clinical* documentation has significant *financial* implications. This is important to remember.

There is a saying, "If it wasn't documented it wasn't done." This is true for medical record documentation. There are situations when audits on medical record documentation may occur, and incomplete records are the kind of unforced errors practices can't afford. Medical records are documents that may be used for legal purposes; inaccurate depictions of a patient's conditions and care could put a practice at risk. Also, confirming a complete note prior to claims submission will help reduce the rate of denials and payment recoupments during an audit. To paint a complete picture, the documentation must be comprehensive, legible, and accurate. There are many perspectives from which medical record documentation will be viewed, so painting this complete picture allows for all stakeholders to use this information in a manner in that is relevant to their needs.

Consistently providing detailed documentation promotes quality healthcare, enhances communication between healthcare providers, and captures the level of risk and severity of the patient's conditions. It also demonstrates medical necessity, which is the principal criteria for payment, denial reduction, reduced risk of audit recovery, and ensuring accountability and transparency. It is important to close the loop on problems or conditions identified in the chief complaint and/or managed in the assessment and plan. The problem list in an encounter note should detail medical conditions and illnesses. The level of specificity provided in this documentation will assist with explaining the complexity and severity of illnesses. This in turn justifies code selections and reimbursement.

Patient	Practice Staff	Billing Staff	Manager	Payers
To explain treatment fosters personal care management	Use health information for daily clinical & administrative operations	Enables accurate billing & collections for improved revenue	Offers baseline for compliance & risk mitigation	Provides necessary data for claims adjudication & payment

Figure 7.1   Stakeholders' Use of Medical Record Documentation

Quality documentation will demonstrate the results of treatment and the patient's progress, or lack thereof, with a medical necessary treatment plan. This also include medical rationale for decision making for orders such as labs, radiology, surgery, and DME. Providers should be cautious when using abbreviations and acronyms to be sure that the reader of the note can understand, within any context, the information documented.

Every encounter note must be able to stand alone; meaning that one shouldn't need to search other resources in the chart to understand what occurred in a visit. Providers should ensure that the original note clarifies and justifies that rendered services are accurate and medically necessary. Today, even with electronic records systems, most organizations still chart in a Subjective, Objective, Assessment, and Plan (SOAP) note format. This format reviews *subjective* observations, *objective* observations, provides an *assessment*, and dictates a treatment *plan*.

This layout typically begins with the chief complaint, gathering a history of present illness (HPI), moves into the review of systems (ROS), and then concludes with the assessment and plan (A&P). The benefit of the SOAP note layout is that most providers are familiar with this method of documentation. In fact, most providers will automatically scroll to the bottom of another provider's note on the assumption that the A&P is at the bottom. This note layout is also conducive to the clinical workflow, as the items covered represent a natural method of review in the exam room.

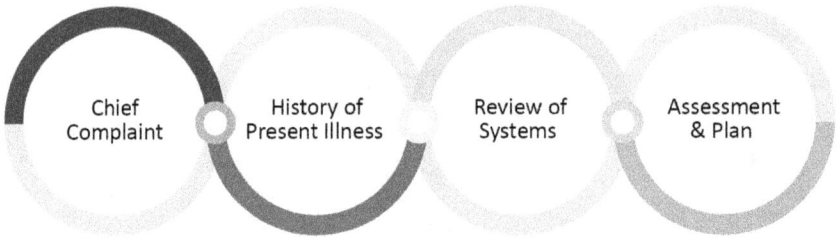

| Chief Complaint | History of Present Illness | Review of Systems | Assessment & Plan |

Figure 7.2   SOAP Note Format

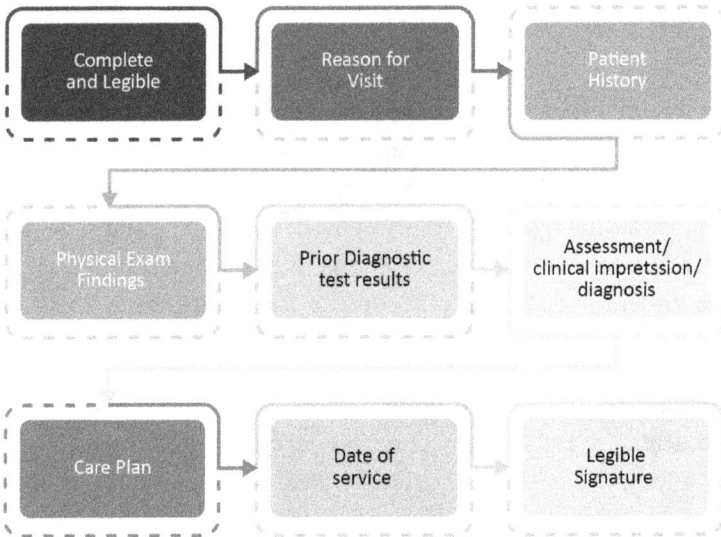

| Complete and Legible | Reason for Visit | Patient History |

| Physical Exam Findings | Prior Diagnostic test results | Assessment/ clinical impretssion/ diagnosis |

| Care Plan | Date of service | Legible Signature |

Figure 7.3   Medicare's Medical Record Documentation Guidance

There are many guides to consider when formatting documentation. Providers participating in the Medicare program should be aware of and follow Medicare's medical record documentation standards. Practices using an EHR will have an easier path to compliance with these standards, as certified EHR's have programmed many of these functions, capabilities, and templates. As you customize your EHR visit encounter

140

templates, consider using Medicare's documentation guidance as a baseline for clinical documentation.

Charting on Paper

There are providers who may prefer to document on paper without the use of EHR technology. Practices who opt to use paper medical records and meet the MIPS participation criteria will incur a MIPS financial penalty. Providers who take a paper/EHR hybrid approach to documentation may ask their clinical staff to just scan in their handwritten notes into an EHR. This process circumvents direct data entry and direct data capture, which reduces reportable data for quality payment programs. This negatively affects auto-coding assessments, quality program financial incentives, note legibility, and clinical-decision support tools. Using manual and paper processes deducts from a practice's return on investment (ROI) for the EHR, creating additional and expensive duplicative workflows. Paper records also create higher levels of vulnerabilities for risk for security, privacy, and timeliness of orders, care, and claim submission.

EHR Benefits, Frustrations, and Vulnerabilities in Documentation

In 2015, a small practice was dealing with a large power outage due to a blown transformer nearby. Luckily, the practice had many windows and, with emergency lighting, was able to keep the practice open during daylight hours. The providers were both clinical and academic and researchers at heart. The wealth of data at their fingertips, thanks to discrete data analytics in EHRs, was immeasurably valuable to them and, yet, when they heard the announcement that they would need to chart on paper, they applauded. It may seem contradictory that clinicians with an ingrained love of data diving would be happy to not have access to the system that accumulates that data for them, but it's a wonderful example of the love-hate relationship many practice staff have with EHRs.

EHRs come with obvious benefits: notes can be templated and prepopulated with known patient information, referrals and refills can be sent with the click of a button, and patient data is being amassed and consumed at unprecedented rates. Now that so much data is at our fingertips, we have the added responsibility to ensure that this data is reviewed and addressed. This double-edged sword requires active data management. As an example, a practice has a lab interface for orders out/ results in. If patients' lab results are not electronically sent to the physicians' EHR inboxes for review prior to the patient's appointment, this will result in the physicians being unaware of findings. Although a physician will be able to locate the results, gaps in care may occur in this instance if results, tests, and other pertinent medical information are not properly managed.

The frustrations in using EHR technology sometimes seem to outweigh the benefits from the clinician's perspective. This is an important point for managers and administrators. When clinicians are frustrated with constant mouse-clicking and incessant patient account alerts, they look for workarounds and solutions that improve their personal workflows. It's important to work with clinicians and establish a platform for feedback that is genuinely received and, where possible, implemented.

When clinicians begin developing their own software system workarounds, it can create a host of issues with documentation and coding based on the impact of pre-programming within the software. Additionally, missing system capabilities may provide encouragement for other bad habits. Testing clinician software use experience during implementation will proactively identify issues and provide an opportunity for corrections. Check in with clinicians regularly on their EHR user experiences to optimize use of an EHR. A clinician's EHR experience directly impacts accurate and complete documentation.

Effective use of EHR for Medical Record Documentation

Under current standards, practices interested in participating in the MIPS program must utilize a certified EHR to be in compliance under the Advancing Care Information category, and to qualify for bonuses under the quality category. Check here to see if your EHR is "certified EHR technology" (CEHRT): https://chpl.healthit.gov/#/search. Notably, CEHRT status, like records documentation and payments, may be audited and rescinded. Stay abreast of current software version availability, CEHRT status, and payment program regulations.

Procedure codes (CPTs and HCPCS) and diagnosis codes (ICDs) are updated annually. Consider keeping track of these updates; connect with your EHR vendor to ensure that your software contains the most up-to-date code sets from a reputable data source. During EHR implementation, based on the practice specialty, it's also a good idea to create short lists or quick lists of commonly-used diagnosis and procedure codes and to educate all users to avoid confusion on code searches. Template development is another key to completeness and medical record documentation accuracy. An appropriately-documented medical record can reduce many of the hassles associated with claims processing and may serve as a legal document at some point in the course of care to verify elements and outcomes of care provided. All practice staff who are performing data entry, document management, or visit notes should be required to ensure accuracy of information.

Cloning Documentation

The term *cloning* refers to the copying and pasting of patient information from one note to another. For example, a provider may elect to have the HPI or ROS automatically pull in from the previous visit for today's visit. When this happens, it is easy for providers to skip a review and edit of these sections in the note. Thereafter, it's impossible to determine if the provider in fact reviewed and assessed the patient in a manner consistent with key factors necessary based on medical necessity.

Cloning notes may also result in over-documentation and regurgitating old or unrelated information. For example, cloning a statement like, "Mrs. Jones is a 50-year-old female who smokes 2 packs of cigarettes a day." Once the patient turns 51 years old, and the provider is still pulling in old data, this will create an inaccurate new note. You also want to be sure that the cloned information is relevant and is addressed in the current visit. If it is not being addressed in the current visit, it is not helpful to be included. For auditing purposes, cloned documentation is increasingly seen as reason for payment reviews and recoupments.

Over-Documentation and Upcoding

Often EHR systems can auto-code the notes based upon the documentation. In some EHRs, the system even identifies the factors required for higher-level coding. The intention originally was to give providers insight into appropriate coding and to provide ongoing education. Unfortunately, in some cases, what it taught providers was that the inclusion of additional information, whether irrelevant or unnecessary, may be beneficial from a payment perspective.

Appropriate use and documentation are the goals. If items documented are outside the chief complaint, unrelated to the visit, and unnecessary or exaggerated, they may represent over-documentation to upcode the visit to a higher reimbursement level. Formulate and customize EHR note templates and cloning rules during the EHR implementation phase. When developing templates, it is necessary to educate providers on how best to utilize note templates to avoid single clicks without reviewing and editing prior to saving. There are instances when check boxes may not be appropriate or require fine-tuning to fit each unique encounter.

Pre-Charting/Pre-Coding

Some providers may pre-complete their charts or coding to save time. Completing the record or coding for the visit prior to it occurring is not appropriate. Completing the note prior to the visit increases the likelihood of the inclusion of errant information in the record. In a normal situation, with documentation performed during or immediately after the visit, blank spaces in the note remind the provider to review that section. In a pre-completed note, there is no reminder to the provider, so areas for review can be missed, erroneous information may be left in the note, and critical updates may not be documented.

Encounter Note Close Out

With the many obligations and activities vying for a provider's time and attention, providers may fail to document visit notes as soon as possible.

You should look for creative and engaging ways of encouraging providers to complete notes in an accurate and timely fashion.

Medicare discourages delayed medical record documentation and considers a documentation timeline of 24 to 48 hours as "reasonable." Factoring the number of unique patient visits one provider will perform on a given day, it is challenging for a provider to remember with accuracy all pertinent details of each unique visit without timely documentation. Medicare could consider documentation timelines outside of these ranges as being unreasonable. Since Medicare is used as an industry benchmark, consider using this guidance in your practice when developing documentation and chart locking protocols.

COMPUTER   If your EHR supports it, consider setting a time limit for when charting is locked. Combine that with an alert to management and providers who can be pro-actively prompted to follow-up for review, completion, and sign-off. A reactive but effective opportunity to leverage technology in the process of medical record documentation oversight is to run "unlocked medical record" reports. This data will allow you to identify encounter notes that have not been locked to send reminders to the provider to close the note. This information may also be used to cross reference claims filings for locked or unlocked notes.

There are resources to assist providers with automating and expediting the medical record documentation process, including voice recognition software, scribe services, and customized EHR apps and tools. CMS has tasked each Medicare Administrative Contractor (MAC) with policy setting for their respective regions. Urge providers to seek guidance in understanding participating payer and Third-Party Administrators (TPAs) medical documentation requirements.[1]

TPAs: Third-Party Administrators act as the processing group on behalf of another entity. For example, let's say Cutten Mend Health Insurance provides coverage across three states. They process claims in two states, but in the third, they outsource claims processing to another company, Processed4U. In this case, Processed4U is the TPA of Cutten Mend Health. Patients are insured and covered by Cutten Mend Health, but all processing documentation (claims, EOBs, ERAs, and other correspondence) will be sent to and from Processed4U.

1995 vs 1997 E&M Documentation Guidelines

E&M code guidelines are based on criteria created by CMS. There are two sets of documentation guidelines, 1995 and 1997; one published in 1995 and the other published in 1997 (hence the 1995 / 1997 nomenclature). Notably, E&M codes are under review for significant legislative change, so stay up-to-date about proposed and/or newly finalized regulations regularly to stay abreast of potential E&M coding changes.[2] The proposed changes may impact the manner in which key documentation components are used to score and attain CPT® levels and may place more emphasis on medical decision making and time as components for CPT® level selection.

Providers should select the guidelines that best fit their documentation needs and that are advantageous. The examination is the major difference between the two guidelines; using the 1995 guidelines allows a provider to more easily attain a comprehensive exam, which in turn may impact the overall CPT® level. Many providers prefer using 1995 guidelines, as the examination is left to their discretion. Using 1997 guidelines involves required components within the examination that in many instances are beneficial for use by specialist providers who are focusing on a specific body system. It is recommended to use one documentation guideline per encounter.

> COMPUTER Check with your EHR vendor to determine your template customization options based on the 1995 or 1997 guidelines you wish to use. It's also a good idea to determine which guidelines your software is using for automated encoding within the medical records.

Excerpt from 1995 / 1997 Documentation Guidelines

Medical record documentation requires the recording of pertinent facts, findings, and observations about an individual's health history including past and present illnesses, examinations, tests, treatments, and outcomes. The medical record chronologically documents the care of the patient and is an important element contributing to high quality care.[3]

Medical Coding

Much emphasis has been made on accurate and complete encounter documentation. Let's delve into medical coding, which is the interpretation of healthcare visit notes, procedures, medical testing, laboratory services, surgeries, procedures diagnoses, equipment, and drugs. The interpretation is converted into alpha-numeric codes. On a basic level, coding from medical record documentation includes interpreting the following data and converting it into the following structures:

Table 7.2

Medical Record Data	Code Interpretation
Illness, Injury, Condition, Health Status, External Causes	ICD-10-CM
Services, Procedures	CPT®, HCPCS
Procedures, Supplies, Products, Services	HCPCS

These codes have many uses. Below are a few of the most common uses:

1. By providers of care: they often do not have specialized training but get on-the-job training; they do the best they can to understand the complex rules of documenting services and applying codes to those services.

2. By the EHR: most have an encoding capability that allows for automated code selection based on the templates used and documentation presented. After completing documentation, the EHR will recommend codes for the provider to select or the provider may choose to code manually.

3. By certified coders: educated and certified individuals who must earn a certain number of continuing education credits and stay up to date with industry coding changes to remain certified. Certified coders interpret providers' documentation and determine appropriate code selections.

Evaluation & Management Documentation Guidelines

A good starting point with E&M documentation guidelines is to distinguish a new patient from an established patient. This is important because there is a higher level of work attributed to treatment of a new patient, which in turn increases the level of Relative Value Unit (RVU) and reimbursement. CPT® rules may not completely match payer guidelines, so always cross-reference both for proper code selection.

New Patient

CPT® defines a new patient as one that has *not* received care within the past three years from the same provider or another provider of the same specialty and belonging to the same group practice.

In the case of a covering provider, just because they have never seen the patient, they are not automatically permitted to bill a new patient service. A covering provider must bill for the same services that the original provider would have been eligible to bill.

Two providers in the same specialty may not both bill new patient codes for the same patient within the three-year time period.

The term *same specialty* is an important factor, because if a provider's taxonomy code is listed incorrectly, this may impact the manner in which new patient codes are billable. The taxonomy code is also a factor for new patient rules within incident to guidelines. To start, the physician must initiate the care plan for a new patient for incident to designation. If the physician refers a patient to a mid-level provider of a different specialty and taxonomy code, then the mid-level provider may bill as a new patient service.

Established Patient

CPT® explains that an established patient *has* received care within the past three years from the same provider or another provider of the same specialty and belonging to the same group practice.

If a provider either has multiple TINs or leaves one TIN to join another group TIN, any patients seen by that provider under the prior TIN within the past three years will not be considered new patients under the new TIN. Example: A physician employed by a hospital leaves the hospital to open a private medical practice. Patients who have been seen by the physician at the hospital wish to follow the physician and be seen at the private practice six months later. Since the patients have been seen within the three-year threshold by the physician (as indicated via the reported NPI) the services would not be billable as new patients.

For extended guidance on distinguishing new from established patient coding guidelines, please refer to the latest CPT® manual.

E&M Components

E&M coding includes a scoring system that is used to determine the CPT® code and level selection. The scoring system is comprised of components that make up the actual E&M services that are performed by healthcare providers. These components should be documented accurately for proper service code selection.

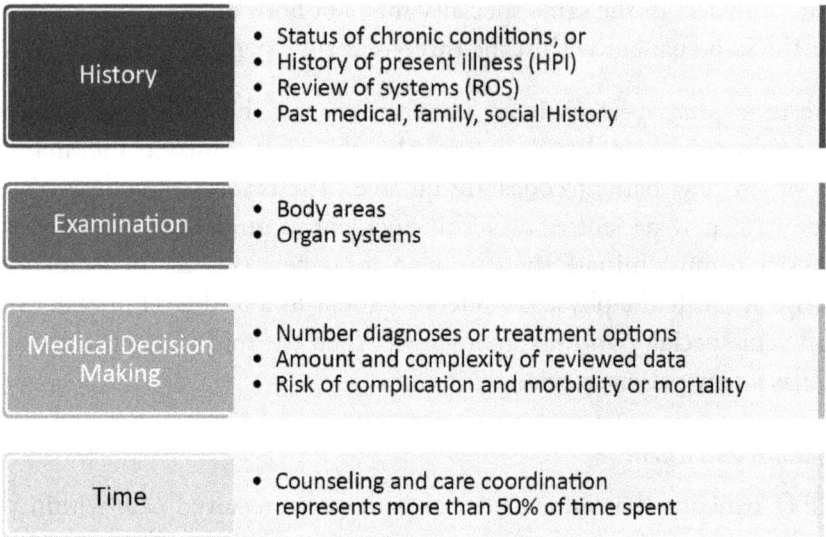

Figure 7.3   Key E&M Components

Each component listed above comes with specific requirements and expectations that comprise the overall score and ultimately determine the CPT® code level. These expectations will be well known and understood by individuals who have received specific training and certification in coding practices. It is important to note that the rendering provider *must* personally record the HPI. This is the only history element that should not be recorded by ancillary staff.

E&M New and Established Patient Scoring

The final options for scoring History and Examination elements are:

- Problem Focused (PF)
- Expanded Problem Focused (EPF)
- Detailed (D)
- Comprehensive (C)

The final options for scoring Medical Decision Making (MDM) by level of risk, which in turn provide the level of complexity, are:

- Straightforward (SF)
- Low Complexity (L)
- Moderate Complexity (M)
- High Complexity (H)

New Patient CPT® Scoring[4]

	Three elements are required in a column to achieve the CPT® level, or the CPT® level will be downgraded to the left.				
History	PF	EPF	D	C	C
Exam	PF	EPF	D	C	C
MDM	SF	SF	L	M	H
Avg Time	10 min	20 min	30 min	45 min	60 min
CPT® Code	99201	99202	99203	99204	99205

Established Patient CPT Scoring[5]

	Two elements are required in a column to achieve the CPT level, or the CPT level will be downgraded to the left.				
History		PF	EPF	D	C
Exam		PF	EPF	D	C
MDM		SF	L	M	H
Avg Time	5	10	15	25	40
CPT Code	99211	99212	99213	99214	99215

Code Categories

Access to the code categories below is available through different ways. Two of the most common sources used to access codes are annually published coding books and search engines within EHRs. These code categories include:

Current Procedural Terminology (CPT®)

This code set describes many of the medical services, surgeries, and procedures conducted by healthcare providers. The American Medical Association (AMA) owns the copyright to CPT® codes and updates and publishes these codes on an annual basis.

To better understand the use of CPT® codes, it is helpful to understand essential medical terminology, including prefixes, suffixes, root terms, and anatomy. Depending on your practice's specialty, there will be certain categories that are more pertinent to your area of medicine. It's a good idea to become familiar with that category and obtain resources to stay up to date on changes, innovations, and trends.

Examples of body systems and CPT® code categories are listed below:

Category II Codes

This code category is not a required component for reimbursement. These are "tracking codes which facilitate data collection for the purposes of performance management. Capturing this data helps to drive Health Effectiveness Data Information Set (HEDIS) performance improvements."[6]

HCPCS Level II

HCPCS is a collection of codes and descriptors defined to represent procedures, supplies, products, and services. These codes are then used to communicate that information to Medicare or private health insurance to describe what beneficiaries and enrollees experienced during their visit.

Evaluation and Integumentary	Anesthesia	Surgery
Integumentary System	Musculoskeletal System	Respiratory System
Cardiovascular	Digestive System	Urinary System
Male Genital	Female Genital	Nervous System
Eye and Ocular Adnexa	Auditory System	Radiology
Pathology and Laboratory	Medicine	

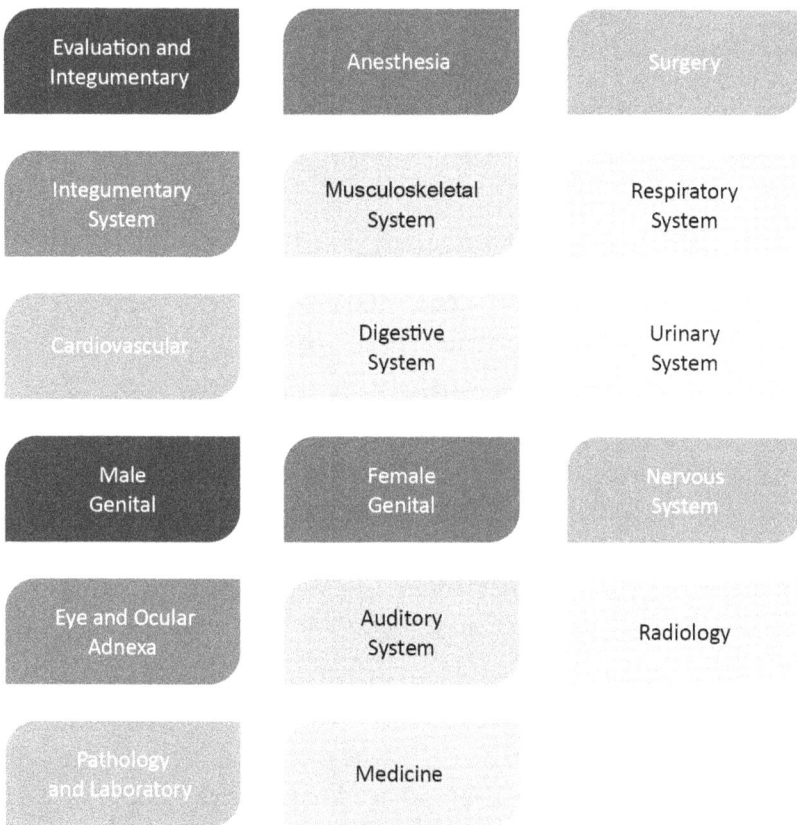

Figure 7.4   Examples of Body Systems

ICD-10-CM

ICD refers to the classification of diseases in a codified data set; ICD-10 refers specifically to the 10th edition of this code set. While there are a few practices today still using ICD-9, the currently required edition is the 10th edition. The biggest change from ICD-9 to ICD-10 is the level of specificity available in the code set. ICD-10 codes are updated regularly, and billing staff should ensure all coding updates in EHRs and PM systems are quickly implemented. When managing diagnosis code selection, be on the look-out for overutilization of unspecified codes. With the conversion to ICD-10-CM, code specificity is available and should be used to accurately explain conditions and illnesses.

Nurse Visits

Nurse visits are becoming more frequent as regulations and expectations increase. There are specific requirements for face-to-face nurse visits which are billed as CPT 99211:

- *This is for established patients only.*
  - Do not report code 99211 for services provided to patients who are new to the physician/practice.
- *The provider-patient encounter must be face-to-face.*
  - For this reason, telephone calls with patients do not meet the requirements for reporting 99211. According to CPT®, the staff member may communicate with the physician, but direct intervention by the physician is not a requirement.
- *An E/M service must be provided.*
  - Generally, this includes a review of the patient's history, a limited physical assessment or some degree of decision making. If there is no clinical need then, 99211 is not appropriate. For example, 99211 would not be appropriate when a patient comes into the office just to pick up a routine prescription.

Consultation Codes

Since 2010, Medicare does not pay physicians for consultations using the CPT® consultation codes; however, some commercial payers will reimburse for these services. Check your payer fee schedules and provider manuals to determine consultation code reimbursement guidelines. CMS increased the work relative value units (wRVUs) for new and established office visits to accommodate the elimination of consultation code reimbursement. Clinicians should instead report the CPT® codes (99201 – 99205) for New Patients or 99212-99215 for Established Patients) depending on the complexity of the visit. Use E&M code descriptions to find the appropriate match.

Consult Codes – Three Year Rule

Examples of where a new patient office visit is <u>not</u> billable

(taken from the Medicare Learning Network Provider Inquiry Assistance article Revisions to Consultation Services Payment Policy – JA6740[7]):

- If the consultant furnishes a pre-operative consultation at the request of a surgeon on a beneficiary, and the consultant has provided a professional service to the patient within the past three years, then this situation would not meet the requirements to bill a new patient office visit.

- The consultant could not bill for a new patient office visit for a consultation furnished to a known beneficiary for a different diagnosis than he or she has previously treated if the patient has seen the consultant in the prior three years.

- The consultant furnishes a consultation to a known beneficiary in an outpatient setting different than the office (e.g., emergency department) observation where the patient has seen in the past three years. As the patient has seen the consultant within the past three years, a new patient office visit is not appropriate.

Prolonged Service Codes

As healthcare providers are being urged to prevent exacerbations, minimize hospital admissions, prevent unnecessary emergency room visits, and coordinate care, patient visits are becoming lengthy. With this rise, the use of prolonged service codes may be appropriate. Prolonged service codes should be billed along with the base E&M code. Medicare has provided time thresholds for each code. The first hour should be billed with CPT 99354, with additional 30-minute increments billed with CPT 99355 following the first hour of prolonged services. CPT® codes require documentation that supports the time being billed; this is especially true when billing prolonged service codes. Prolonged services are add-on codes and do not require a modifier, as they are only applicable when being reported with an appropriate E&M service.

Table 7.3   Prolonged Services Thresholds[8]

E/M CODE	AVERAGE TIME	99354 THRESHOLD TIME	99354 & 99355 THRESHOLD TIME
99201	10	40	85
99202	20	50	95
99203	30	60	105
99204	45	75	120
99205	60	90	135
99211	Nurse Visit	n/a	n/a
99212	10	40	85
99213	15	45	90
99214	25	55	100
99215	40	70	115

Time-Based Coding

There are three components to consider when the decision is made for time-based coding

1. Document the total time of the visit.

2. State that more than 50% of visit was spent counseling or coordinating care.

3. Clearly document counseling or coordination of care content.

Coding Compliance

CMS is a federal agency within the U.S. Department of Health and Human Services (HHS) that administers the Medicare program and works in partnership with state governments to administer Medicaid. CMS is one of the largest purchasers of healthcare in the United States.

"Medicare is the second-largest program in the federal budget. In 2018, it cost \$582 billion — representing 14% of total federal spending."[9]

National Correct Coding Initiative

> The CMS developed the National Correct Coding Initiative (NCCI) to promote national correct coding methodologies and to control improper coding leading to inappropriate payment in Part B claims. The CMS developed its coding policies based on coding conventions defined in the American Medical Association's CPT Manual, national and local policies and edits, coding guidelines developed by national societies, analysis of standard medical and surgical practices, and a review of current coding practices. The CMS annually updates the National Correct Coding Initiative Coding Policy Manual for Medicare Services (Coding Policy Manual).[10]

Ideally, medical practices should attempt to download or integrate the annual NCCI edits into their EHR/PM software. This permits flags or alerts when incorrect coding or documentation has occurred, and therefore would provide an opportunity to correct any issues. It's always a good idea to check with your EHR/PM software vendor regarding interfacing capabilities.

In order to remain compliant, providers should understand all documentation and coding guidelines applicable to the services they provide. Most out-patient physician practices utilize E&M CPT® codes. Educating providers can be done through internal programs or through outsourced programs, regardless the important part is that the education is completed.

Monitoring Provider Utilization of E&M Codes

Medicare and other payers will benchmark E&M utilization data in the form of a bell curve chart. In these charts, frequency of utilization is plotted vertically, and code levels are plotted horizontally.

Bell Curve Data

As named, ideally the plotted units by level will be in the shape of a bell. This tool provides a very quick method of spot-checking providers' E&M coding.

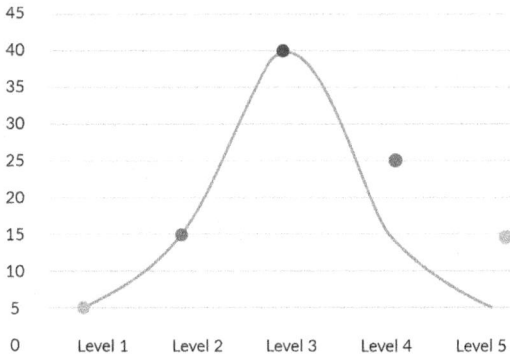

Figure 7.5   Sample Bell Curve

In this assessment, the center of the bell should be in the center of the graph. A bell curve with the center far to the right may indicate inappropriately high coding. A bell curve with the center too far left may indicate the opposite. To assess for your practice, AAPC has a bell curve simulator that compares your data, as you enter, to national Medicare benchmark utilization data for your specialty (https://www.aapc. com/resources/em_utilization.aspx).

Who Should Audit Documentation?

This is a challenging question. Auditing documentation is time-consuming, and the resulting necessary corrective actions can be frustrating and complex, but the overall process is vital. There is value in having peer-to-peer audits where providers review one another's documentation. The challenge with this approach is that the providers' understanding of documentation and coding guidelines and standards will vary, jeopardizing the accuracy of final results. So how do you audit provider documentation? The first step is to identify high-risk areas and assess whether this is something you can manage in-house or whether it would be prudent to outsource to an expert.

There are pros and cons to both solutions, usually with the best solution being a blend of the two options. Best practice is to maintain an internal program with a regular schedule for assessment. Scheduling reoccurring audits should be done based on risk areas and applicable corrective actions. Audits should be performed bi-annually or annually. Below are a few differences between in-house and outsourced coding audit programs to get your thought processes started:

Table 7.4   In-House versus Outsourced Auditing Program Assessment

In-House Audit Program	Outsourced Audit Program
Staffing	
Burdensome regulations and required processes often leave minimal availability to consistently accomplish with existing staff who have other responsibilities. Many practice staff do not have training in coding.	External entity should be certified and up to date in all related guidelines and regulations. They would communicate audit results to practice staff for implementation. External entity could develop internal audit processes, protocols, and controls to provide this guidance to practice staff.
Cost	
Many think the cost to perform in-house is non-existent. This is not true; you should still evaluate the hours required for staff to complete the audit, investigate unfamiliar rules, validate findings, create provider training, and develop processes against total compensation. Also factor in possible downtime in other work duties, such as claim submission and A/R follow up for the individuals doing the work performing the audit.	Depending on the vendor, the cost to perform an audit would be based on several factors, including: Number of encounters being reviewed, number of providers included in the review, amount of data being reviewed, electronic access or the requirement of being onsite, and past performance. Obtaining a flat rate would bundle all expenses as opposed to an hourly rate, which could become costly.

Bias	
Individuals regularly performing audits on the same providers may begin to get audit fatigue and miss or accept commonly seen errors. This is a challenge unique to internal entities that become accustomed to provider documentation habits.	Outside organizations attempt to remain free of bias when evaluating records but may face a different challenge. Some practices believe that only individuals at their practice understand the unique needs of their specialty/facility/patient base, etc. and will devalue the recommendations of the outside entity.
Education	
When performing internal audits, it is the responsibility of the facility to ensure staff have the knowledge and skills to perform documentation audits. Where there are deficiencies, the facility should offer the opportunity for the staff to obtain additional education or training in documentation auditing. Educating the providers is an essential component of an audit program. Providing regular provider education on trends and specialty updates is essential.	Confirm the training and education styles, mechanisms, and resources for each vendor to ensure alignment with providers learning needs. It is recommended that external entities use certified resources to conduct training programs. Some practices may look to obtain CMEs for education; the process and cost should be considered. The practice is better served including education into a bundled cost for the overall external audit.

As a practice administrator, manager, or executive, it isn't within your scope to provide clinical guidance or to assume any kind of medical decision making. It is your responsibility, however, to ensure that documentation is accurate, complete, reviewed, and audited, and that guidance and education for continuous documentation improvement is implemented within your practice. Documentation auditing may be performed internally or may be outsourced to a third-party. The key is to make sure that the individual performing the assessment and education is knowledgeable (preferably certified) and that they are providing appropriate critique and guidance to your clinical staff and providers based on NCCI, CMS, commercial payer, and specialty-specific guidelines.

Auditing Resources

Practices that elect to audit documentation internally should reference reputable and accredited resources for support. Relying on sources that nationally recognized for setting standards, advocating for improvements and those that offer certifications add to the legitimacy of internal audit results. Organizations that set documentation and coding best standards include:

- American Health Information Management Association (AHIMA)
    - ○ This national industry leader in health information management has many resources, including relevant certification programs and educational resources.
- AAPC
    - ○ This national organization is a leader in proper coding, documentation, and auditing practices. AAPC has several coding certifications and has expanded to other relevant certifications.
- Centers for Medicare and Medicaid Services (CMS)
    - ○ CMS has become a benchmark for payers, hospitals, providers, and administrators across the nation in many ways, including documentation. For guidance on documentation requirements, navigate to www.cms.gov and search the term "documentation guidelines."
- The National Committee for Quality Assurance (NCQA)
    - ○ This organization is focused on the improvement of healthcare quality and provides guidance on documentation best practices for value programs.
- The Institute for Healthcare Improvement (IHI)

     o This organization provides a host of resources including guidelines, processes, workflows, and document templates to improve all areas of practice and clinical management, including documentation.

Other beneficial resources to consider include in-person and on-demand training sessions through accredited organizations like MGMA. Obtaining coding guidance from specialty-specific medical associations allows providers to obtain best practices from their medical specialty subject matter experts. These organizations typically stay on the cutting edge of their specific specialty in medicine and often advocate for positive improvements in that area of specialty. Local medical societies also play a role in ensuring providers have the resources needed for compliance.

What to Look for in Coding Reviews

Auditing metrics and KPIs will vary by facility but common factors for review include legibility, consistent reflection of patient identifiers, provider's signature, and evidence of comprehensive clinical documentation. Other factors to consider in the audit would be to validate codes paid are justified by documentation. This would include comparing services billed with services paid and cross-referencing an auditor's feedback on clinical documentation improvement (CDI). Benchmarking internal providers to one another, as well as to regional or national best practices, is helpful to determine successes and areas for improvement. Trending results over time is also helpful in identifying improvement areas.

An audit should include a comprehensive review of medical record documentation that supports code selection and reimbursement levels. Below are a few examples of areas within medical record documentation that may be reviewed during an audit:

1. Ordering testing without stated intentions in the assessment and plan.

2. Impressions, intentions, findings, and patient status clearly stated within the assessment and plan.

3. Cloning resulting in errors or inconsistencies in HPI, ROS, or PFSH.

4. Medication management, including prescribing of new medications.

5. Addressing the chief complaint within the visit.

6. Complete documentation of history, examination, and medical decision making to justify the CPT® code level.

7. Adherence to prolonged services, preventative services, and time-based coding guidelines.

8. Typos, and also patient age or gender mismatches within the encounter note.

9. Electronic signature is an indication that the provider truly reviewed the note.

10. A hypertension diagnosis with no blood pressure recording.

11. A diabetes diagnosis with no blood sugar or A1c reading.

12. Inclusion of diagnoses that were not addressed during the encounter.

13. Missing diagnoses or lack of specificity in diagnoses.

14. Proper sequencing of diagnosis codes: most prominent code should be listed first.

Type of Audit to Perform

Consider the type of audit to be conducted. If you are looking for results post-claim adjudication, then you'll want to perform a retrospective audit. A *retrospective* review would require a practice to submit a corrected claim if a claim was paid incorrectly based on inaccurate documentation and coding. The advantage of a retrospective audit is that claims submission would not be delayed during the audit. Performing a *prospective* audit will allow for a practice to obtain feedback on documentation and coding patterns prior to claim submission, providing the opportunity to submit a clean claim that includes expert feedback. The prospective audit, however, requires claims to be placed on hold while the audit is being conducted, since documentation and coding feedback is given and applied to claims prior to submission.

In the event a risk area or deficiency has been identified, it's a good idea to consider a controlled audit that targets specific factors, such as a specific provider or payer, CPT®, ICD-10-CM, HCPCS, date range, or place of service. When opting to perform a random audit, it's important that the result incorporates encounters that represent the overall population of encounter types. Most practices select between 10-25 encounters per provider for review.

Keep in mind that the documentation goal, as stated before, is to tell a story, at a very basic level, so that others may follow. Medical record encounter visit notes should be able to answer the following questions:

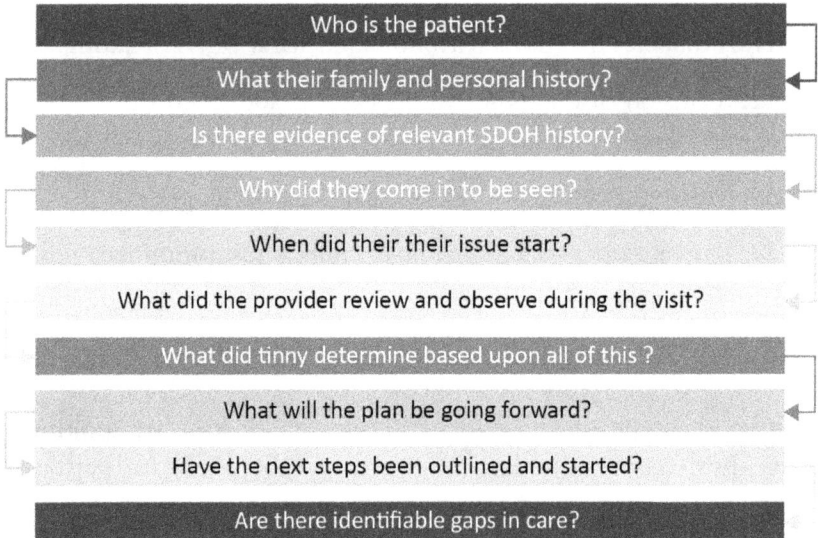

Figure 7.6   Questions to Answer in the Medical Record

At a more complex and meaningful level, additional auditing metrics may be included for purposes of population health. For example, audits on whether (1) a blood pressure reading was taken for all patients, (2) an A1c was drawn and measured for all diabetic patients, or (3) BMI was assessed for all patients. Consider other more specific questions as factors of review during an audit. Set your audit goals to not only include individual patient record reviews but population reviews that will improve overall quality care and quality measures for Advanced Payment Program reporting.

Recovery Audit Contractors (RACs)

Medical practices are advised to develop internal medical record documentation and coding review programs and education to be sure that rules and guidelines are being followed. Failures in these areas may lead to external audits, penalties, payment recoupment, and even payer participation termination. One external entity that conducts medical record documentation and coding audits are Recovery Audit Contractors (RACs). RACs will review claims after payment has been made.[11] The goals of RACs are to detect and correct past improper payments so that CMS and carriers, fiscal intermediaries (FIs), and MACs can implement actions that will prevent future improper payments."[12] Practices may have external audits performed to prepare for RAC audits and to improve documentation. In both situations, it is imperative to remember that RACs are financially incentivized to ensure correct coding occurs. They are paid to identify problems. The RACs can also go back several years during their audit. Any errors or improper payments can be recouped at that time, with a percentage going to the RAC auditor as payment. For this reason, documentation education and regular internal auditing is very important in every practice.

Practices that have designated a liaison (internal or external) to educate providers, and anyone else involved in medical record documentation, will be ahead of the curve. Whether the resource is internal or external, it's important to have someone provide feedback on Correct Coding Initiatives (CCI), provide clarity on documentation rules, set CDI goals, and conduct coding audits. Corrective actions, CDI monitoring, and reoccurring training are essential aspects of an internal coding audit program.

The feedback from an established internal coding audit program will not only demonstrate a culture of compliance but would also empower providers to become better documenters. If possible, it is helpful to include an individual with a nationally recognized coding certification to assist with maintaining coding and documentation compliance.

"Documentation is only good if the next physician who treats the patient can pick up your record and know exactly what happened."[13] *(Rhonda Buckholtz, CPC, CMPE, CPMA, CPC-I, CGSC, CPEDC, CENTC, COBGC, CRC, CHPSE, Chief Compliance Officer)*

Patient Satisfaction and Continuation of Care

Merit-based Incentive Payment System (MIPS) and Advanced Payment Model (APM) participation includes patient satisfaction as a program measure that is used for reimbursement; therefore, practices should make efforts to improve it. MIPS measures that address patient satisfaction fall under the Improvement Activities category, which is 15% of an overall score.[14] Two of these measures are:

1. Collection and follow up on patient experience and satisfaction data on beneficiary engagement; this includes development of improvement plan.

   a. Activity weighting = High

   b. Subcategory Name = Beneficiary Engagement

2. Collection and use of patient experience and satisfaction data on access; this includes outlining steps for improving communications with patients to help understanding of urgent access needs.

   a. Activity weighting = Medium

b. Subcategory Name = Expanded Practice Access

To view all MIPS measures and determine your practice's participation status, go to: https://qpp.cms.gov/. Assess your practice's performance closely. For the above measures, it would be beneficial to review all areas of patient interactions.

Documentation can impact most measures, including patient satisfaction. For example, let's review a few instances in which documentation creates patient dissatisfaction. In these examples we will refer to Dr. Smith, a member of a group practice with insufficient documentation practices.

- Scenario #1: Jane Summers comes in to see Dr. Smith, but he is on vacation. She is scheduled to see another physician in the practice, but due to the insufficient notes of Dr. Smith, the other physician is unable to provide continuity of care.
- Scenario #2: Bob Jones receives a notice in the mail that an upcoming procedure has been denied by his insurance due to a lack of documentation supporting medical necessity.
- Scenario #3: Dave Williams is admitted to the hospital and consents for the hospital to pull Dr. Smith's record of his care. The records received do not identify all tests previously performed. The hospital has no choice but to subject Dave to testing he has already done, thereby incurring unnecessary costs.

In all these scenarios, patient satisfaction is negatively impacted. In some, additional quality measures (for example, Cost) are also negatively impacted. Like all quality-based measures, performance may affect whether a bonus or penalty is received at the end of the performance period. Reduce surprises at the end of the performance period through proactive measures.

Risk-Adjustment Coding

In 2004, CMS introduced the Hierarchical Condition Category (HCC) concept to predict annual cost per beneficiary. It's no surprise that CMS wants to know how much it costs to treat certain populations. This data is driven by assessing beneficiary demographics, Medicaid eligibility, and health statuses. HCCs anticipate healthcare costs of care per beneficiary based on demographics and diagnosis coding. Other factors are also included, for example, if the patient is in treatment for ESRD, institutionalized or residing at home, and if they have dual Medicare and Medicaid eligibility.

Risk-adjustment coding is the use of HCCs to weigh illnesses by severity to assign higher value for higher risk conditions. This is referred to as a Risk Adjustment Factor (RAF) score.[15] This means that an accurate assessment of HCCs is a direct factor of risk accuracy. Since risk is used to assess prospective cost, HCCs have far-reaching impacts and implications. If providers are not accurately documenting illnesses to the highest level of specificity, then an accurate level of risk is not captured, reported and forecasted. This inaccurate prediction will impact payer funding, which will trickle down to provider reimbursement by inaccurate depiction of a patient's health status, outcomes, and disease burden. For example, an inaccurate RAF could give the impression that a provider is managing a low risk pool of patients that may not be deserving of a higher level of reimbursement based on the reported lower risk.

This again echoes the need for provider education on documentation and specificity best practices. Avoid the use of unspecified diagnosis codes as much as possible. The ICD-10-CM code sets provide a wealth of specificity related to illnesses and injuries. Work with billing staff or auditing staff to help catch unspecified codes and return them to the providers for education on proper coding and assignment of appropriate specificity.

Best practices for HCC review and use within the private practice include:

1. Review problem lists in EHR and compare to assessment and plan.

2. Revise outdated unspecified diagnosis codes in a problem list to more specific codes.

3. Address illness and injury coding at each unique encounter.

4. Correct any provider documentation inefficiencies.

5. Support a culture of overall specificity.

6. Document co-morbidities, complications, and manifestations.

7. Regularly audit medical record documentation.

8. Engage Transitional Care Management (TCM), Chronic Care Management (CCM), preventive services, consistent patient engagement and other hospital readmission reduction methods.

9. Understand practice and providers' cost of care ratings.

HCCs are a factor of reimbursement for many value-based payments models and coordinated care models such as Accountable Care Organizations (ACO) and Clinically Integrated Networks (CIN), as well as many insurance payers.

HCC Cost of Care

As the industry moves from FFS to value-based reimbursements, the overall cost of care has become increasingly important. Assess eligible clinicians on their ability to manage the cost of care, which is a risk-adjusted measure, and consider higher cost benchmarks when caring for higher risk populations. Cost of care is also becoming a factor in provider compensation.

As mentioned, the MIPS Cost category is 15% of the overall MIPS score for 2019. This category extracts data from submitted claims to provide cost data and is comprised of ten cost measures. Below is the CMS description[16] of two cost measures that are relevant to most providers:

The Medicare Spending Per Beneficiary (MSPB)

This measure evaluates solo practitioners and groups on their spending efficiency and is risk-adjusted to account for patients' risk profiles. The combination of an NPI and TIN are used to identify solo practitioners. Specifically, the MSPB measure assesses the average spend for Medicare services performed by providers/groups per episode of care. Each episode comprises the period immediately prior to, during, and following a patient's hospital stay. [17]

The Total Per Capita Costs (TPCC)

This measure is a payment-standardized, annualized, risk-adjusted, and specialty- adjusted measure that evaluates the overall efficiency of care provided to beneficiaries attributed to solo practitioners and groups, as identified by their Medicare TIN.[18]

✏ Knowledge Check

CHAPTER 7: Documentation & Coding

Question #1:   MDM stands for _____

Question #2:   RACs stand for
_____ , which vary by state

Question #3:   A nurse visit is billed as CPT_____

Question #4:   True or False? Category II codes are not required for reimbursement; they are for tracking purposes.

Question #5:   Name three stakeholders who rely on accurate medical record documentation:

   1.   _____

   2.   _____

   3.   _____

Question #6:   True or False? Recovery Audit Contractors (RAC) are not financially incentivized.

Question #7:   The main difference or unique factor differentiating the 1995 and 1997 guidelines is the _____ component.

Question #8: The Cost Category comprises _____% of the total MIPS score for 2019.

Answers

Q1: Medical-decision-making,
Q2: Recovery Audit Contractor,
Q3: 99211,
Q4: True,
Q5: Payers, patients, referring providers,
Q6: False,
Q7: Examination,
Q8: 15

Endnotes

1. CMS: "Insurer/Third Party Administrator Services" https://www.cms.gov/ Medicare/Coordination-of-Benefits-and-Recovery/InsurerServices/index.html

2. https://www.cms.gov/Outreach-and-Education/Medicare-Learning-Network-MLN/ MLNEdWebGuide/Downloads/97Docguidelines.pdf

3. https://www.cms.gov/Outreach-and-Education/Medicare-Learning-Network-MLN/ MLNProducts/Downloads/eval-mgmt-serv-guide-ICN006764.pdf

4. https://www.novitas-solutions.com/webcenter/content/conn/UCM_Repository/uuid/ dDocName:00004966

5. Ibid.

6. http://www.e-mds.com/what-are-cpt-ii-codes-and-how-are-they-used-medical-billing

7. https://www.cms.gov/Medicare/Medicare-Contracting/ContractorLearning Resources/Downloads/JA6740.pdf

8. https://www.cms.gov/Outreach-and-Education/Medicare-Learning-Network-MLN/ MLNMattersArticles/downloads/mm5972.pdf

9. https://www.pgpf.org/budget-basics/medicare

10. [www.CMS.gov - NCCI – 12.13.18]

11. https://www.cms.gov/Research-Statistics-Data-and-Systems/Monitoring-Programs/ Medicare-FFS-Compliance-Programs/Recovery-Audit-Program/

12. CMS.GOV – https://www.cms.gov/Research-Statistics-Data-and-Systems/Monitoring-Programs/Medicare-FFS-Compliance-Programs/Recovery-Audit-Program/

13. Book quote provided by: *Rhonda Buckholtz, CPC, CMPE, CPMA, CPC-I, CGSC, CPEDC, CENTC, COBGC, CRC, CHPSE, Chief Compliance Officer*

14. https://qpp.cms.gov/mips/quality-measures

15. https://www.aafp.org/practice-management/payment/coding/hcc.html

16. Taken directly from https://qpp.cms.gov › mips › explore-measures › cost https:// qpp.cms.gov/mips/explore-measures/cost?py=2019

17. Taken directly from https://qpp.cms.gov › mips › explore-measures › cost https:// qpp.cms.gov/mips/explore-measures/cost?py=2019

18. Taken directly from https://qpp.cms.gov › mips › explore-measures › cost https:// qpp.cms.gov/mips/explore-measures/cost?py=2019

Chapter 8

Charge Entry

The practice has registered, scheduled, verified, checked-in, seen, and documented the patient encounter! Now it's time to bill for the professional services rendered, and this process starts with charge entry. Charge entry is the interpretation of medical record documentation converted into descriptive code sets which explain the services rendered, supplies given and conditions treated. This information is compiled into a healthcare claim that will be submitted to the funding source, in our case an insurance company; for reimbursement. *Charges* are the set fees attributed to each service provided. Most professional charges are converted into CPT and HCPCS codes.

Depending on the workflow, it is either the providers or the clinic staff who enter charges. To submit a claim to a funding source, an accurate charge must be created, reviewed, and then released most likely through a clearinghouse to be sent to the insurance company.

Encounter note completion and charge entry should be an overlapping process. Think about it, if the charge is entered prior to the note being completed charges might be missed even still, conditions might not be communicated. It is a best practice for providers to complete the encounter notes for their patients prior to charge entry. The sooner the note is closed and completed, the better. It's best to close notes within

48-hours from the date of service. This allows the provider to remember key points of the encounter and gives staff an opportunity to prepare charges for claim submission.

> When programmed, most EHR/PM software will extract diagnosis and CPT® codes from the progress note, using a process called "encoding." This data is then pulled into a pre-claim window for review, scrubbing with necessary corrections and electronic submission. Be sure to confirm your practice's Charge Description Master (CDM) and applicable fee schedules are correctly uploaded, as this information will be retrieved and used for coding and reimbursement purposes. Capturing accurate CPT® codes starts with the data from a practice's CDM. Many EHR/PM software packages utilize an external database that integrates and maps data to the EHR/PM software to include such elements as clinical terminology, diagnoses, procedures, and much more. This process allows for applicable information interchange, creating an interoperable EHR/PM software. Check with your EHR/PM software vendor to determine which cross-mapping tool is used for your system. Systematized Nomenclature of Medicine-Clinical Terms (SNOMED CT) is one example of a terminology resource for encoding of healthcare terms for electronic health records.

Pros and Cons of Notes-Based Encoding

When utilizing the encoding function of EHR/PM software, take into consideration the pros and cons of allowing the software to do the work for you. Although we want to leverage technology to be efficient, we also do not want to completely remove the provider from the decision-making process of describing and coding of medical services.

PRO	CON
Diagnoses and procedure codes connect to the descriptors in the provider notes, which can reduce the omission of charges.	Using computerized algorithms may result in under- or over-coding for services.
Encoding can identify errors in modifiers or multiple charges prior to submission.	Organizations can become reliant upon encoding and become lax about auditing.
There is typically no additional fee for this feature.	Encoding may result in over-standardization by inaccurately missing variables that could change visit complexity, resulting in duplicative code selections.

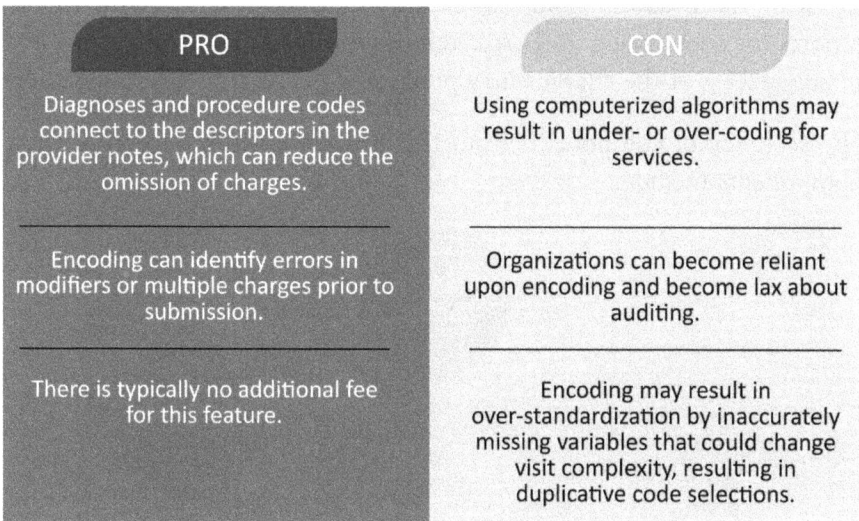

Figure 8.1   Pros and Cons of Notes-Based Encoding

Charge Entry Considerations

Accuracy is a key component of charge entry. Ensuring that patient demographic and insurance information is accurate is integral to avoiding payment denials, incorrect patient balances and communicating a precise health status for each patient. A process that requires reviewing insurance verification details during the charge entry process allows for the confirmation and correction of key patient demographic and insurance information prior to claim submission. Since accuracy is such an important part of the charge entry process, it's also important to consider who in your practice would be responsible for this important task and ensure that they have the resources, time, and skill set necessary for the task. For those responsible for the charge entry function, it is best that they are given time to work uninterrupted without distractions during the process to avoid mistakes.

A checklist of data elements required during charge entry may assist with standardization of the process, thereby increasing the volume of clean claim submission. Leveraging an EHR/PM software to run reports for monitoring and cross-referencing information may also add to the success of the charge entry process.

The accuracy of components from the visit are critical. Several of these components include:

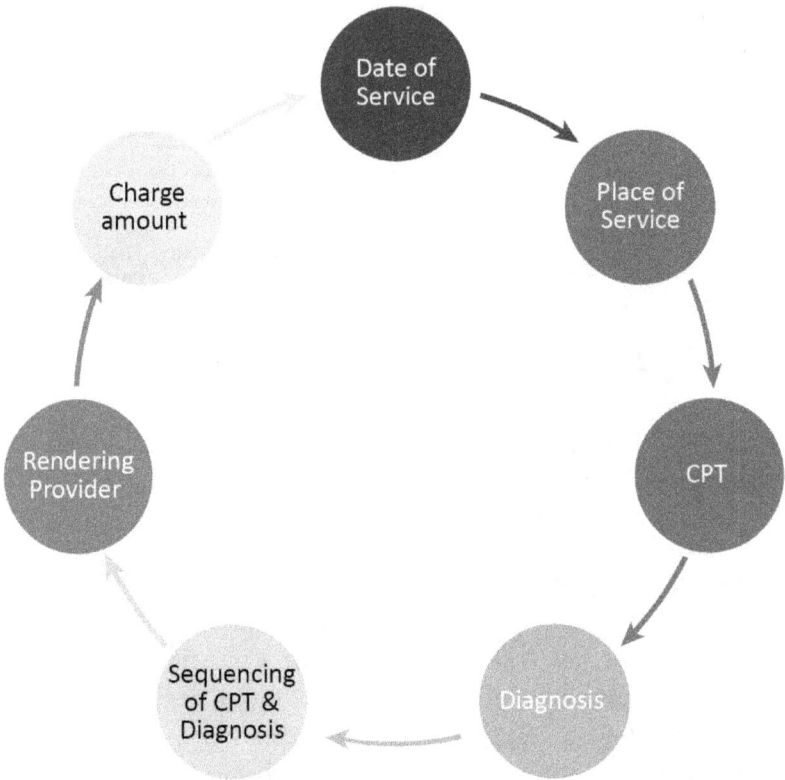

Figure 8.2   Components of the patient visit where accuracy is critical to clean claims submissions

Types of Charges

With the number of unique and qualified services, it is expected that there are varying types of charges. Many medical practice services are considered professional services and will fall under the "Diagnostic and

Therapeutic" services category. Below is a list of commonly used charge types.

- Diagnostic and Therapeutic charges
    - ○ These charges are usually given a flat rate based on a payment formula.
    - ○ This is typically most of a private practice's charge list.
- Time-Based Charges
    - ○ Certain CPT® codes allow for the consideration of time as part of the service, such as, prolonged E&M services, surgical time, and anesthesia.

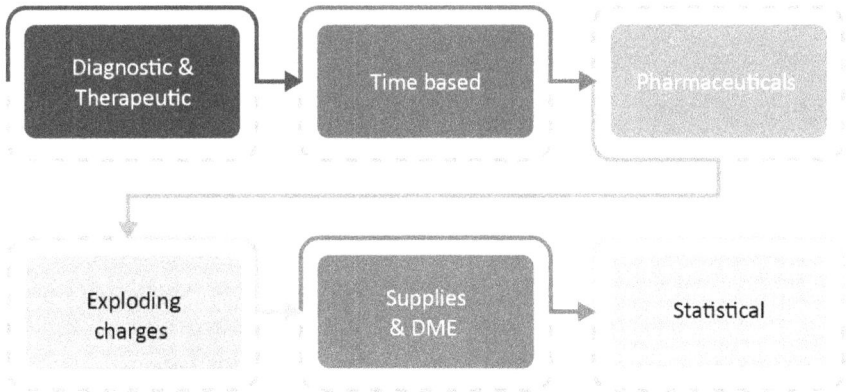

Figure 8.3   Types of Charges

- Pharmaceuticals
    - ○ This will include certain drugs that may be part of the service, including vaccines and other injectables.
- Exploding Charges
    - ○ Permanently grouping certain services codes that are normally billed together in a specific sequence on a claim that are hard coded within the CDM.

- Supplies and DME
  - ○ Payer reimbursement guidelines may differ regarding billable items. These codes are categorized in HCPCS Level II.
- Statistical
  - ○ Some charges are used for informational or tracking purposes only. These will not have a dollar amount associated with them. These codes are categorized in CPT® Category II and Category III.

During charge entry there are several key steps which ensure accuracy of financial information and inclusion of all rendered services. Those steps include:

Step One: Reconciliation of Services to Charges

At the conclusion of services, there should be a reconciliation of services to charges process. Clinical staff, the providers, or any qualified member of the organization may perform this reconciliation. The goal of the reconciliation is to ensure that all services performed are on the charge sheet or superbill before it goes to the billing staff for claim submission. When using PM software for billing, utilize a "missed charges" report to reconcile missed and kept appointments. In the event that a patient missed an appointment, be sure that no rendered services were documented for that date of service. Some version of charge reconciliation should be conducted regardless of whether charge submission is electronic or paper. If your practice uses a HIPAA-compliant sign in sheet during the check in process, after a patient is checked in remove their signature/name sticker from the sign in sheet and place it on a reconciliation document. At the end of the day, that document should have the names of all patients seen on that day. Use that document as a cross-check to be sure all services and monies balance at the end of the day.

Step Two: Code Over-Reads

During the charge entry process by clinical staff, or non-billing personnel, a code selection over-read process should occur. This process should include a review of CPT®, HCPCS and diagnosis codes to ensure accuracy compared to encounter visit notes. Some codes exclude others, some require extra modifiers, and so forth.

> To capture all services, run a report from all machines used for testing and patient care (i.e., spirometry, EKG, echocardiogram, labs). You can then cross-reference these reports with service slips or kept appointment reports to ensure no charges are missed. This allows the practice to verify services were rendered and post applicable charges. Example: A physician completes a patient encounter for shortness of breath and recommends that the patient obtain a pulmonary function test (PFT). The physician forgets to check off the PFT codes for billing on the superbill and the respiratory therapist misses the charges at the end of the day. Running a report on the PFT machine and providing it to the charge entry staff would have avoided the missed charges.

Use of modifiers in conjunction with CPT® codes is another element to consider when preparing charge entry for claim submission. Unless certain modifiers will be used 100% of the time, it is not recommended to hard-code modifiers into a Charge Description Master (CDM), as usage rules may change by payer and NCCI edits.

For these reasons, it is important to have a certified coder or billing expert who can perform a deeper review of code selection and rules for accuracy prior to claims preparation and submission. Designate a qualified individual within the organization to perform these reviews. You can help the practice ensure compliance with guidelines and submission of clean claims by providing this person with additional resources, such as:

- Access to annual coding updates
- Specialty specific coding guidelines
- Payer reimbursement guidelines

Step Three: Posting Patient Payments

If the process has not had copayments posted during the check-in process, monies collected by patients should be posted during the charge entry process. It is important to document patient payments as soon after receiving as possible to show an accurate picture of the patient's account. Posting copayments properly will make it clearer to close claims after insurance adjudication. If not, the patient may receive an invoice for a payment they've already made or, they may receive an invoice for a copay that states they also have a credit in the same amount. Both situations can make the practice look disorganized and can foster frustration in patients.

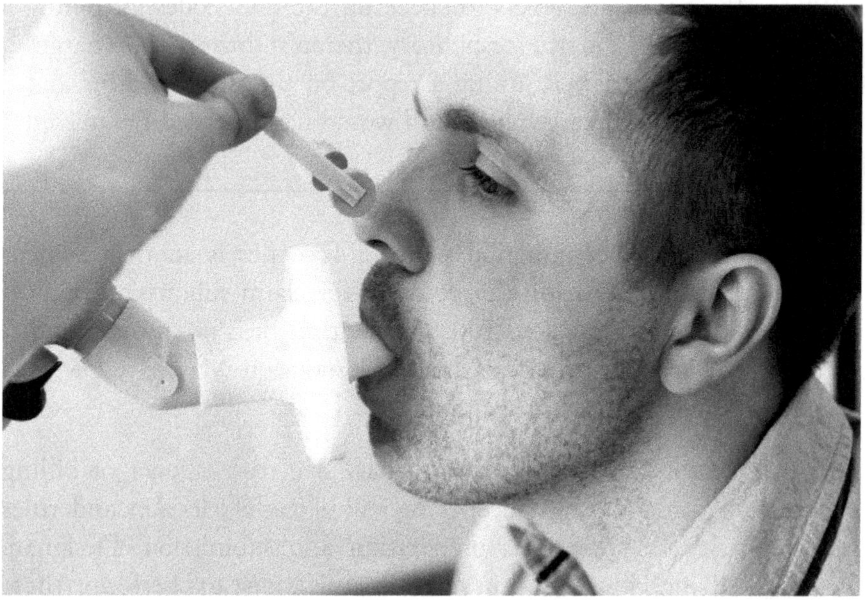

Figure 8.4

In the event a patient payment is posted incorrectly and results in an overpayment, start an investigation to research the validity of the overpayment. There are services that, based on the patient's insurance benefits; a copayment may be waived. An example could be a physical exam or some other preventative service. In this case, if the practice may be unaware of a waived copayment and one is collected from the patient at the time of service resulting in an overpayment. It's best to wait until the claim is fully adjudicated to determine the validity of an overpayment before refunding the patient. Once a patient overpayment is confirmed, the patient should be notified and refunded immediately. If the patient has an upcoming appointment, consider giving them the option of applying the credit toward their upcoming visit. If they decline that option, send them the payment in the manner your practice uses for accounts payable (i.e. check, secured bank transfer, etc.).

Step Four: Data Entry

When it's all said and done, charge entry boils down to accurate data entry. Knowing and accurately applying key data points is the foundation of charge entry. This data entry requires the utmost accuracy. It's important to avoid duplicate charges by reviewing a patient's account prior to initiating a new claim.

Special Considerations for Advanced Practice Clinicians (APCs)

There are considerations to be made when processing claims for Medicare that include the services of qualified non-physician providers (NPPs). By using the following information when processing those claims, NPP services can be reimbursed at full fee schedule value rather than the 85% reimbursement you would usually receive from Medicare. Commercial payers may, but not always, adopt the Medicare standards as their own. Check with individual payers for their reimbursement guidelines.

Supervising Provider versus Rendering Provider

Claims require documentation of the supervising and rendering provider. In some cases, this is the same person; in others, it is not. The supervising provider is the provider overseeing the provider who performed or "rendered" the services. Again, the rendering provider is the provider who performed the services.

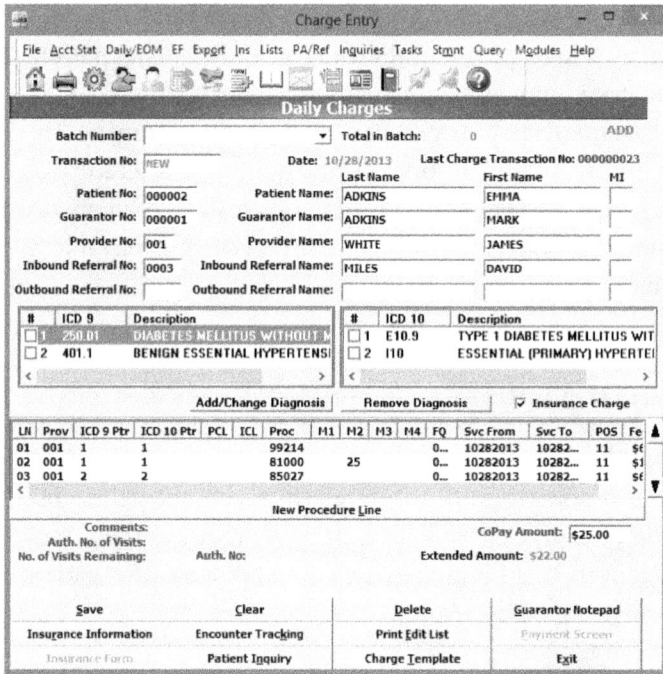

Figure 8.5   Charge Entry window in American Medical Software
Source: *https://www.softwareadvice.com/resources/how-icd-10-software-helps-at-transition-stages/* [1]

Some states do not require a supervising provider for certain mid-level providers, so check state and insurance carrier guidelines on the required relationship between certain supervising and rendering providers. In the event a supervising provider is required, a collaborative practice agreement (CPA) might be necessary. The CPA will outline the scope of practice for the provider who requires supervision along with the supervision expectation by the supervising provider. Many practices will include this CPA as a point of employment and basis of insurance credentialing for mid-level providers. The necessity of a CPA should be confirmed by your state medical board.

Incident-to Billing

Incident-to billing (a Medicare term) is common for advanced practice clinicians (APCs)[2] or as some consider "mid-level providers," who bill under the NPI number of a supervising physician in an outpatient setting. When incident-to billing guidelines are met, the services performed by the APC are paid under the supervising physician's NPI number at 100% of the supervising physician's allowable amount.

> To qualify as "incident to," services must be part of your patient's normal course of treatment, during which a physician personally performed an initial service and remains actively involved in the course of treatment. You [the physician] do not have to be physically present in the patient's treatment room while these services are provided, but you [the physician] must provide direct supervision, that is, you must be present in the office suite to render assistance, if necessary.[3]

For example, if a Physician Assistant (PA) sees a patient in the office, they would be the rendering provider for that visit. The physician on-site, supervising the PA, is the supervising provider.

There are rules that are applicable to billing services as incident-to a physician's professional services:

1. The physician must perform the initiating new patient visit and establish the care plan.

2. The physician must remain part of the treatment process; patients should not only see an APC throughout the course of treatment.

3. The care provided by the APC should relate directly to the treatment plan laid out by the physician. The APC should not create new treatment plans or address new problems without the physician's supervision. New treatment plans would include new diagnoses or illnesses that will be treated in addition to those established by the initiating physician.

4. The physician should remain onsite and available to the APC during the visit encounter.

5. The individual furnishing incident-to services must meet any applicable requirements to provide such services, including licensure imposed by the state in which providers render services (i.e., physician assistant, nurse practitioner billing Medicare under the physician's NPI).

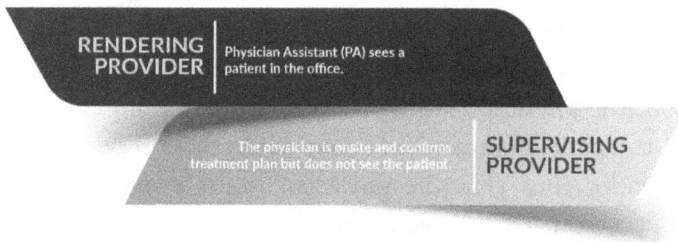

RENDERING PROVIDER — Physician Assistant (PA) sees a patient in the office.

The physician is onsite and confirms treatment plan but does not see the patient. — SUPERVISING PROVIDER

Figure 8.6   Rendering Provider versus Supervising Provider

You will want to keep an eye on regulatory changes and CMS interpretation for incident-to billing as this is a frequently misunderstood and misused concept. Other incident-to billing policies, rules, and regulations may vary by payer. You will want to make sure you and your staff are up to date on rules before billing incident-to services. In lieu of incident-to billing, the APC may check with the insurance carrier's guidelines and move toward becoming a credentialed participating provider under their own NPI number, not requiring physician supervision. Credentialing APCs directly with insurance companies gives the APC the ability to initiate care plans and treat new patients so that they may bill for services directly to the payer instead of under the supervising physician. Medicare will reimburse the APC or eligible NPP 85% of the CMS allowable amount.[4] Again, each payer has unique APC reimbursement guidelines, so it's best to research prior to initiation of billing.

Place of Service

CMS maintains the Place of Service (POS) code set, which are two-digit numeric identifiers meant to represent the location service was provided. Different POS codes will be reimbursed at different rates by Medicare and Medicaid, as well as commercial payers. There are just under 100 POS codes.[5] The POS documented on the claim will determine which codes to use and the reimbursement amounts that apply. It's vital that the POS code being used for services is accurate. This should be established under practice settings in your PM software during customization. Common POS codes are:

02 - Telehealth

11 – Office

13 – Assisted Living Facility

15 – Mobile Unit

19 – Outpatient Hospital (Off Campus)

20 – Urgent Care Facility

21 – Inpatient Hospital

22 – Outpatient Hospital (On Campus)

23 – Emergency Room Hospital

24 – Ambulatory Surgery Center (ASC)

26 – Military Treatment Facility

31 – Skilled Nursing Facility

50 – Federally Qualified Health Center

72 – Rural Health Clinic

The CMS webpage will have the most current POS code set, though it is published many places. Be sure to review the full descriptions, as some have exclusions.[6] For example, the POS 11 is for offices, but not offices located in community health centers, skilled nursing facilities, or hospitals. Make sure to select the correct POS during charge entry.

Telehealth

HealthIT.gov defines *telehealth* as "the use of electronic information and telecommunications technologies to support and promote long-distance clinical health care, patient and professional health-related education, public health and health administration."[7] This form of treatment is increasing in popularity especially in rural areas or areas of provider shortage.

> LIGHTBULB Health professional shortage areas (HPSAs) are areas where there are not enough providers (health, dental, medical, etc.) to meet the needs of the population for that area. To identify HPSAs, navigate to https://data.hrsa.gov/tools/shortage-area/hpsa-find. Operating a practice in an HPSA may open your facility to additional reimbursements or support systems funded by HHS and other federal/state agencies.

Depending on the insurance payer, telehealth services may have very specific requirements. With most commercial insurers, patients who have telehealth coverage can use a commercially available telehealth platform. These platforms allow patients to connect with available providers within minutes, process their insurance and submit their copayment.[8]

This can be an excellent stream of ancillary revenue for providers, as long as telehealth hours do not detract from face-to-face onsite visits and all requirements are met for documentation and billing.

Billing Telehealth

It is important to review the guidelines, per payer, prior to performing and billing telehealth services.[9] Some payers allow telehealth services to originate from any location. Others, like Medicare, require the originating site to be an HPSA or an MSA (Metropolitan Statistical Area). These services include audio visual appointments delivered via computers and smartphones.

Through telehealth services, the patient can see and hear the physician, who is able to see and hear the patient as well. For rural patients, patients without transportation capability, or even those that are just stuck at work, this is quite a useful service. Regardless of the payer, the POS on telehealth claims is 02.

> For more information on Medicare's telehealth requirements, navigate to www.cms.gov and enter the search term *telehealth*.

Remote Care Management

This category of services includes services such as Chronic Care Management (CCM) and the non-face-to-face portion of Transitional Care Management (TCM) services. Like telehealth services, remote care management services are for patients who are not onsite with the provider. *Unlike* telehealth services, remote care management services use video less often in favor of telephone or electronic communications. The POS should match the location that the provider would ordinarily deliver services; no special modifier required.

CPT® codes identify remote care management services instead of POS codes. Additionally, some payers include a list of designated remote care services for which their beneficiaries are eligible to receive care.

Common remote care management services include:

- 99091 Remote Patient Monitoring (RPM)
  - ○ This involves the monitoring of patient data through wearable devices or the transmission of that data from one technology to another for review.
- 99490 Chronic Care Management (CCM)
  - ○ This involves the ongoing management of patients with multiple chronic conditions in excess of 20 minutes per month.
- 99487 Complex Chronic Care Management
  - ○ This is like CCM, but the time and complexity requirements are higher.
- 99495/6 Transitional Care Management (TCM)
  - ○ These codes are related to the management of patients post-discharge or during other points of transition in care.
- 99492-4 & 99484 General Behavioral Health Integration (BHI)
  - ○ These codes relate to the management of behavioral health conditions in team-based formats. [10]

Confirm insurance coverage and benefits prior to providing services and discuss any patient responsibilities in advance of services.

Chapter 8 Knowledge Check

Charge Entry

Question #1:

True or False?   Advanced practice clinicians should initiate a new patient visit for an incident-to service.

Question #2:

True or False?   Exploding Charges are hard coded within the CDM to group certain service codes that are normally billed together in a specific sequence on a claim.

Question #3:

Match the following Place of Service (POS) codes with their description:

11	Urgent Care
13	Assisted Living Facility
20	Office
21	Ambulatory Surgery Center (ASC)
22	Inpatient Hospital
24	Outpatient Hospital (On Campus)

Answers

Q1: False

Q2: False

Q3: 11=Office, 13=Assisted   Living Facility, 20=Urgent Care; 20=Inpatient Hospital, 24=Outpatient Hospital (On Campus)

Endnotes

1. https://www.softwareadvice.com/resources/how-icd-10-software-helps-at-transition-stages/

2. Medicare refers to APCs as *non-physician providers* (NPPs), and the US Department of Justice's Drug Enforcement Administration (DEA) uses the term *mid-level practitioner* for their own purposes. We feel *advanced practice clinicians* or APCs is the best and most respectful way to refer to providers in this category of direct treatment of patients. Until there is widespread standardization, it is in everyone's best interest to clarify what leadership includes, even within their own practice.

3. MLN Matters – CMS #SE0441 (https://www.cms.gov/outreach-and-education/medicare-learning-network-mln/mlnmattersarticles/downloads/se0441.pdf)

4. https://med.noridianmedicare.com/web/jeb/topics/incident-to-services

5. https://www.cms.gov/Medicare/Coding/place-of-service-codes/Place_of_Service_Code_Set.html

6. https://www.cms.gov/Medicare/Medicare-Fee-for-Service-Payment/PhysicianFeeSched/Downloads/Website-POS-database.pdf

7. https://www.healthit.gov/topic/health-it-initiatives/telemedicine-and-telehealth

8. https://www.healthit.gov/topic/health-it-initiatives/telemedicine-and-telehealth

9. https://www.cms.gov/Outreach-and-Education/Medicare-Learning-Network-MLN/MLNMattersArticles/downloads/MM10393.pdf

10. https://www.cms.gov/Outreach-and-Education/Medicare-Learning-Network-MLN/MLNMattersArticles/downloads/MM10393.pdf

Chapter 9

Claims Preparation & Submission

The claim submissions process is how claims get to the insurance companies for payment. Most claim submission processes today are automated. Previously physicians could just write down what services they provided, write down an amount to pay, and send that over to the insurance company, which would then pay that exact amount. Then the process required the submission of a paper HCFA, but today, claims are submitted by electronic means. Luckily for us, the automated claims process has made claim submission much easier for practices.

The basic first step is to make sure you list the most current information on the claim during initial submission. This definition is for a "clean claim," meaning it contained no errors. Denial prevention starts with a clean claim.

It is also important to include any additional required documentation. For example, you will want to include required referrals or authorizations with the claim. Where indicated, include medical records documentation as well, or make a process to submit this documentation with all claims as a standard operating procedure.

Failure to submit a clean claim the first time can result in processing delays or even non-payment. Appropriate preparatory processes help ensure the submission of clean claims. The claims preparation process should include review of the superbill, claim generation, manual scrub, submission to the clearinghouse, and review of the claims edit report.

Review of Superbill

The superbill has had many names over the years: fee ticket, visit fee sheet, or fee slip. Regardless of terminology, the purpose is the same: to capture the services provided and diagnoses assessed for each patient seen for claims generation.

Paper superbills typically look like the document in Figure 9.1:

	CPT	Description	ICD-10	Description	
Patient Name: Jane Doe			**Acct #: 12345**		
DOS: 1/1/2021			**Provider: [} Smith [X] Jones**		
	99202	NP Visit Level 2	E11.9	Type 2 Diabetes Mellitus w/o Complications	
X	99203	NP Visit Level 3	E78.5	Hyperlipidemia (unspecified)	X
	99204	NP Visit Level 4	E03.9	Hypoactive Thyroid (unspecified)	X
	99213	F/U Visit Level 3	D64.9	Anemia (unspecified)	
	99214	F/U Visit Level 4	110	Essential (primary) Hypertension	X
	96372	Injection Administration			

Figure 9.1   Example Superbill

The superbill doesn't include all the chart notes. It should, however, include the information necessary to identify and bill the services rendered. Some superbills are more comprehensive and include full patient demographics. Other superbills have less information than the example above, maybe only including on-site testing (i.e., pulmonary function testing).

The superbill is meant to be a customized document reflecting the most frequently used procedure and diagnosis codes for your practice.

Superbill Utilization

These days, most practices have moved to electronic charting and, often, these systems will support auto-coding or automatic claims creation (see Chapter 7 for more information on auto-coding). Even with automatic claims creation, much of the industry still refers to paper superbills as a final check against the documented services rendered.

Superbills support many needs. They are useful to confirm charge entry for all patients seen by ensuring there is a claim for every patient seen. They can also be utilized to confirm that charges entered include all services rendered, ensuring that there is a charge for everything billable performed during the visit.

Superbills are also useful as a comparison tool. For example, billers can check diagnoses on the superbill against diagnoses documented in the chart. For prompt payment, billing requires the use of the most specific and appropriate diagnosis codes, so it is important to check these codes for errors. It is vital to discourage the use of catch-all codes like "not elsewhere classified." Superbills can also be used to review cash copay collections for the patients who were seen. (See more about this in Chapter 10.)

Of the above, the most common uses are the first two, which confirm charge entry for *all* services performed on *all* patients seen. It is worthwhile to manually review each superbill against each claim and verify that each procedure is documented on both. If there is a discrepancy, refer to the provider's documentation or reach out to the actual provider for confirmation.

Manual Scrub

Some practices still submit CMS-1500 paper forms. Practices that use PM systems use the electronic claim version of the CMS-1500, called the 837P. The majority of private practices submit claims electronically (837P) via a PM system.

PM systems serve as an electronic database that houses patient demographic information, as well as historical appointment and billing information. Integrated PM and EHR systems may auto-generate and auto-code claims.

After claim creation, perform a manual scrub. A manual scrub is a process where a reviewer looks at certain details of the claim to prevent submitting a claim with an obvious error. The reviewer(s) should:

- Compare procedures and diagnoses to those listed in the chart (unless performed previously).
- Review procedures for appropriate use (some procedure codes may exclude others listed).
- Review modifiers listed to make sure they match up to the services performed and that required modifiers are present.
- Look for Medically Unlikely Edits (MUE).
- Make alterations to align with individual payer reimbursement guidelines.
- Look for CPT® mismatch.

Keep track of errors found in the scrubbing process for the provider and staff education. Submission of a clean claim is critical to the RCM process; the manual scrub is a vital step in this process.

Required Attachments

After appropriate claims documentation, attach pertinent information to the claim. Whether that's documentation from the visit, referrals, authorizations, lab results, (or anything else that would be critical toward substantiating payment) attach all required documents with the original claim submission. The reasoning is again to ensure that you submit a clean claim. Whether or not the claim was clean will affect the right to payment, appeals deadlines, and total days in A/R.

Accounts Receivable: Amounts in A/R are outstanding balances due payable to the organization. This can include balances due from patients as well as from insurers.

Third-Party Billing Companies

To outsource or not to outsource? That is a question asked quite often. When billing is outsourced to an external agency, that company is referred to as a third-party biller. The choice of whether to use a third-party biller can be difficult to answer because it relies upon factors entirely unique to the practice in question.

Services Offered

External billing companies may offer standard services only or they may offer a whole host of RCM services. Standard services for third-party billers include claims submission, charge capture, denial management, and payment posting. Additional RCM services may include contract management, coding optimization, and overall integrity of the full revenue cycle.

Fees

The fees for third-party billing services vary, but most practices can expect to pay a percentage of receipts. The percentage is typically negotiable, and this is an area practices should discuss and evaluate thoroughly prior to signing any agreements. Percentage-style fees can add-up.

There are also more general fee models that include set monthly rates, per-provider flat fees, and flat fees per claim. Be cautious of third-party billers who offer coding optimization as well as percentage-based reimbursement and closely review their processes, as this method provides an incentive for them to errantly up-code. This doesn't mean that all third-party billers are untrustworthy. If you paid your staff based upon a percentage of collections, then you would want to closely review their code change processes as well. Do not allow your third-party billing company to change codes billed without approval on a claim-by-claim basis from your internal staff.

Management and Oversight

Though outsourced billing services can be helpful in reducing overhead, they will not completely negate the need for internal staff who are knowledgeable in the billing process. Your staff should regularly review claims submitted, missing charges, days in A/R, collections rates, denials, and uncollected amounts.

If you choose to outsource, the oversight of your billing processes should not go away. Though outsourced agencies are not practice employees, they are still responsible to the practice for their actions. If you are considering outsourcing, develop your oversight plan in advance.

The oversight plan should include:

- expectations on communicating errors and denial trends,
- limits on adjustments that are not contractual,
- setting up patient payment plans,
- providing reports back to the practice, and
- structured payment for services that may tie in performance driven measures.

Should I Outsource?

Unfortunately, we can't answer that question for you, but we have listed some considerations in Table 9.1 to think about while making your decision.

Table 9.1 Considerations on outsourcing

	In-House	Outsourced
Cost	Review the total cost associated with hiring billing staff. Include costs for annual training and education updates. Estimate costs for annually purchasing new coding manuals. Is the total cost higher or lower than 6-9% of annual collections?	Review the pricing models for the third-party vendors being assessed. Use a full-year of receipts data to estimate percentage-based costs. Are there add-on fees to consider? Do you need to include costs for the personnel who will oversee the third-party? Are you willing to pay up to 6-9% of your total collections to an outside agency?
Location	Do you have the space to house billing staff? Or do you need to build out additional space?	Where is the company located? Can you sit down for a face-to-face discussion regularly? Are they familiar with the billing regulations and laws of your state?
Services	Do you have the educational resources to manage and train your team in the full RCM?	Are there services the outsourced agency will not perform i.e., tertiary billing services, or credentialing?
Staffing	Do you have any inefficiencies or gaps in your billing processes that cannot be easily resolved? High turnover? Technology barriers?	What are their hiring requirements for staff? Do they have ongoing billing education for staff? Do they perform background checks on employees?
Other Questions	Is your staff cross-trained, or can they be, to cover other positions to minimize stoppages due to staff outages?	Do you prefer full control over the RCM? Is the ability to walk into the billing department to ask questions important to you?

For further guidance on third-party billing compliance, refer to the OIG's *Compliance Program Guidance for Third-Party Medical Billing Companies* by navigating to https://oig.hhs.gov/fraud/docs/complianceguidance/thirdparty.pdf.

Clearinghouse

The selection and use of a clearinghouse is an important function of revenue cycle management. The clearinghouse serves as an intermediary between the practice and the insurance company. To optimize the use of a clearinghouse, there will be a bidirectional interface between the practice's PM software, the clearinghouse, and the insurance company's claims adjudication software. This interface allows for the output and sharing of information between all three parties. There are PM vendors who have established their own clearinghouse that is included in the software.

> SHOUT OUT GUY
>
> As with any third-party vendor, it is important for the practice to perform due diligence before selecting a clearinghouse. Review pricing, fees, capabilities, deliverables, termination policies, and other critical contract terms.

The purpose of the clearinghouse is to help identify potential claim issues before they cause a delay in processing or reimbursement. Optimizing the use and oversight of the clearinghouse can have significant benefits to the practice including faster claims processing, better coding utilization, more detailed reporting, and an overall shorter claims cycle as shown in Figure 9.2.

After claims generation, preparation, and manual scrubbing, submit claims to a contracted clearinghouse. Once the clearinghouse receives the claim, they will scrub the claim electronically with their software to check for errors and to verify the claim format is appropriate for the insurance payer. Since the clearinghouse transmits claims to payers, they will also be aware of and can provide guidance on payer claim edits for corrections to avoid payment denials.

Clearinghouse Interface Flow
What path does the claim take?

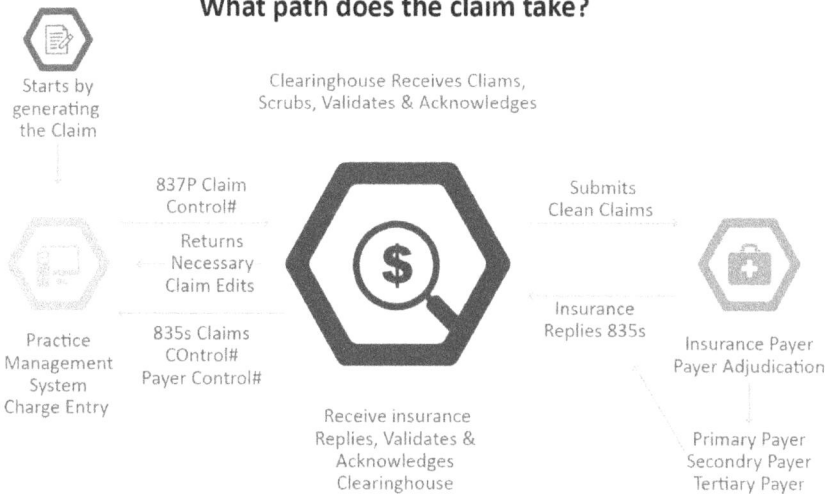

Starts by
generating
the Claim

Clearinghouse Receives Cliams,
Scrubs, Validates & Acknowledges

837P Claim
Control#

Submits
Clean Claims

Returns
Necessary
Claim Edits

Practice
Management
System
Charge Entry

835s Claims
COntrol#
Payer Control#

Insurance
Replies 835s

Insurance Payer
Payer Adjudication

Receive insurance
Replies, Validates &
Acknowledges
Clearinghouse

Primary Payer
Secondry Payer
Tertiary Payer

Figure 9.2   Clearinghouse Interface Flow

Claims Edit Report

Clearinghouses will automatically generate claims edit reports to provide feedback on potential claims submission issues. This communication gives the practice the opportunity to correct any claims errors, to submit clean claims the first time. The goal would be for the clearinghouse to securely transmit error-free claims to the insurance payers for adjudication and payment. Common claim edit issues include incorrect provider information, place of service mismatches, code or modifier mismatches, and duplicate claims.

Incorrect provider information includes things like missing NPI numbers. Place of service mismatches include many situations. For example, if a hospital procedure code is billed with an 11 POS code, this will require updating the POS code or providing an explanation that verifies the POS originally billed.

Code and/or modifier mismatches are very common. For example, if a claim has a multiple service modifier billed alongside a single CPT® code, it will require a code and/or modifier correction. Another common claims denial issue that a clearinghouse can help a practice avoid would be duplicate claims. To process these, first verify the clearinghouse correctly identified a duplicate claim; then delete the duplicate. Make sure to keep the most comprehensive, accurate, and appropriate claim, regardless of order of creation.

You will want to review claim edit reports daily to avoid delays in the claims process. The greatest benefit of the claim edit report is that it grants the practice an additional opportunity to review the claim and ensure it's clean prior to payer submission.

✎ Chapter 9 Knowledge Check

Claims Preparation & Submission

Question #1:

Failing to submit a clean claim can result in

_____ or _____

Question #2:

The electronic version of the CMS-1500 is the _____

Question #3:

Clearinghouses will automatically generate _____
to provide feedback on potential claims submission issues.

Answers:

Q1: delayed payments or denied claims
Q2: 837P
Q3: Claims Edit Report

Chapter 10

Deposit Management & Internal Controls

Deposit management consists of all the processes, policies, and audits associated with tracking and reconciling cash, checks, and credit card payments for services rendered. These payments may come through the front desk or from funding sources such as insurance companies. Effectively managing deposits ensures that patients do not receive unnecessary bills for services that they paid but have not yet posted and deposited. These processes are a critical point within the revenue cycle to verify payments are applied to the appropriate services, thereby closing out owed amounts. Depositing payments in a timely manner leads to successful cash flow and patient satisfaction.

Internal controls are an important component of deposit management. These controls can be an easily overlooked area in smaller practices, but they are critical tasks for those interested in reconciliation and preventing fraud and embezzlement in the workplace. Effective internal control policies and procedures will discourage fraud, provide protection to company resources, and maintain compliance with related regulations.

Without including internal controls within a deposit management process, incoming payments through the mail or across the front desk may never make it to the bank.

Cash collections at the front desk should be done in an organized manner. As the front office becomes busier throughout the day, it can become difficult to keep track of payments, especially for organizations that deal with a high amount of self-pay patients. It is essential that practices review money movement throughout the practice and develop internal controls to diminish risk of loss.

Internal Controls

Money can come into the practice through many channels. The front desk takes cash and checks, processes credit cards, and receives mail. The billing department receives mailed payments including checks, credit card numbers and virtual credit cards. The practice may directly receive EFTs from insurance companies into its bank account. Verifying the bank account being used for EFTs and requiring that a corporate check signor is the only individual authorized to finalize an EFT initiation reduces the risk of fraudulent banking activity. The call center/receptionist may also receive credit card payments by phone. Or your practice may allow patients to pay online through a web portal. Additionally, if the practice outsources billing and bad debt, external individuals might collect on the practice's behalf.

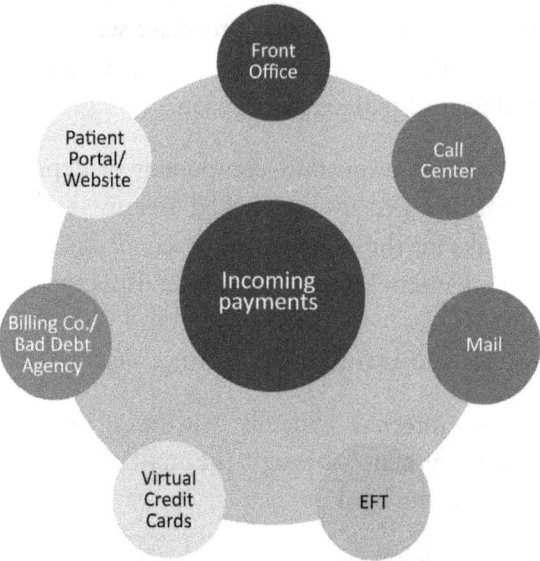

Figure 10.1   Sources of incoming payments

With so many avenues for money to move into the practice, there are equivalent avenues for money to move out. If you have good hiring practices, you may believe that you have very trustworthy staff, and you may very well have trustworthy staff. But it isn't worth testing. The greatest deterrence to theft is removing the opportunity, and the fastest method of discovering theft is through well-structured processes and regular supervision.

Some examples of internal controls to consider:

1. **Reduce the number of individuals who accept payments from patients.**

   a   If patients call in to make a payment, does that number ring all staff or are payments restricted to qualified billing personnel and the front desk? Assigning specific staff to accept telephone payments allows for easier tracking and accountability.

2. **Reduce the number of hands checks pass through.**

   a   When the mail comes in who opens and sorts the mail versus who deposits payments. How many hands do the payments go through prior to posting? Directing all incoming mail related to payments to a specific staff person will give them the ability to report back on mailed insurance payments as well as initiate the EFT process to reduce the number of incoming checks thereby streamlining the revenue process.

3. **Decline to keep credit card numbers on file.**

   a   Unless credit card numbers are in a secure, restricted-access location with careful monitoring of who accesses the information, the practice is asking for trouble. For example, do you keep paper documentation of credit cards in the office? Is it secure? Who has access? Is your PM system able to store credit card information and hide all but the last four digits from general view? Are you able to set permissions to restrict access at the user level? If you decide to keep credit cards on file, ensure that only a portion of the credit card information is visible at any time within your software. This reduces unauthorized use after the initial credit card capture.

4. **Track payments across the front desk by person.**

   a   Is each employee required to balance at the end of the night? Against what are they reviewing? Is there a cross measure that audits this process?

COMPUTER   Many EHR/PM software can track payments posted by user. Consider using this auditing tool for internal tracking. Compare this information to daily receipts used for deposit preparation.

Review the above questions/scenarios against the workflow at your practice to assist in setting up internal controls.

Money Collection

The actual money collection process is one of the largest and easiest opportunities for employee theft to take place. If your front desk receptionist takes in three cash copays, would you know? How can you verify? The answer is process, supervision, and diligence.

Processes that minimize the opportunity for theft, like double-checking cash counts and receipts, are required to remain diligent. Employee theft doesn't just occur with new employees. It can come from long-term employees who are disgruntled or experiencing financial distress and see an opportunity to alleviate a personal problem.

> SHOUT OUT GUY Utilize employee background checks through reputable organizations to look for past civil or criminal offenses that may tie back to financial misdeeds. Employment verifications can also provide insight into past money-handling experience. Include cashier and/or money-handling duties in respective employee's job descriptions. Finally, implement organizational expectations and consequences for failure to follow financial deposit management and internal controls.

As mentioned earlier, copay collections increase when performed during check-in instead of check-out. Staff can be trained to contact patients and discuss past due balances ahead of patients' upcoming appointments. They can also be trained to review past due balances with patients at the TOS.

An end of day review of superbills will confirm accurate copay collection for each patient. If employees batch together the superbills they checked in with corresponding checks, credit card receipts, and cash collected, this provides another assessment of TOS collection.

Audit batches nightly to ensure accuracy and implement internal controls that allow for the separation of duties. For example, the staff person who collects money at TOS should be different from the staff person who deposits the payments at the bank.

No process is going to be 100% theft-proof; where there's a will there's a way. However, the above processes provide a significant deterrent. If a patient's superbill states they have a $20 copay and there is no check, cash, or credit card receipt substantiating receipt of payment, then this needs to be reviewed with the individual who prepared the batch.

Deposit batches should go from the person who collects the cash (generally the front desk) straight to the individual making the bank deposit (generally a manager). Cash goes missing fast, so reduce the number of hands involved and make the cover-up process as burdensome as possible.

Spend some time thinking about the current processes at your organization and how money could go missing. Think about excuses for missing money that you would ordinarily consider acceptable. Put some form of oversight or process on each one. A comfortable or frequently anticipated excuse is an excellent place to hide theft.

Reconciliation Process

After tracking money across the company to the point of deposit, reconcile the deposits through a preset process of checks and balances. This process should include basic balance checks. For example, EFT payments should match corresponding bank deposits, and credit card batch amounts should match corresponding bank deposits. For cash and checks, consider a two-person count with a carbon copy deposit slip. The deposit receipt, carbon copy, and bank deposit should all match.

> SHOUT OUT GUY If, during reconciliation of the monthly bank statements, undocumented deposits are identified, then it's very likely that the billing department is unaware these were received. Under those circumstances, it's important to retrieve payer EOBs from the payer portal. You can then locate the correct deposit by amount and deposit date.

Most payer portals allow you to download the EOB so your billing department can appropriately post payment. Significant delays in posting payments and adjustments can lead to delays in the claim's submission to any secondary and tertiary payers. It can also lead to delays in assessing the patient's balance and getting invoices out to collect any money due from the patient.

If you don't have electronic access to the company bank accounts, then call into the bank's automatic transaction lists or reconcile when the monthly bank statement has been received. Preferably, deposit reconciliation should occur daily. Remember, the sooner you identify theft, the smaller the total loss may be to the practice.

Timing of Deposits

Financial deposits keep a practice's cash flow going, which is why we want to deposit funds as frequently as possible, while keeping in mind the processes it takes to get to the point of deposit. Holding deposits for long periods of time negatively impacts a practice's financial health and will paint a false picture of the status of accounts. Delayed deposits may result in A/R staff continuing attempts to recoup payments for received but not deposited payments. This creates unnecessary work, follow up, investigation, and frustration.

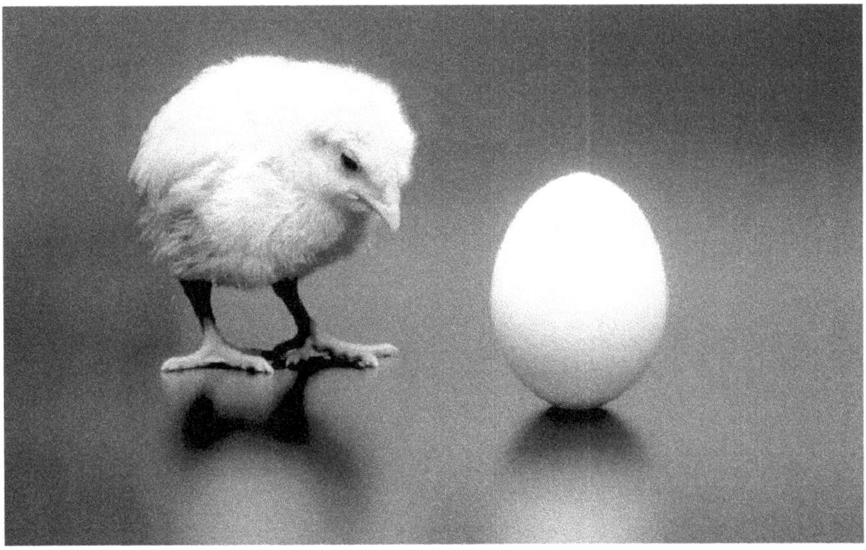

Figure 10.2

There are now electronic banking deposit features that allow for virtual deposits that can eliminate the need to leave the office to deposit funds; this in turn can increase the frequency of deposits.

As you consider when to deposit funds, also think about the timing of payment posting. It's beneficial to have payments deposited prior to payment posting. There might be an urge to get a payment posted right away but fight it; allow the payment to be deposited prior to posting.

Problems may occur when you post a payment prior to funds being deposited. The deposit may not clear. In this case, if the payment was posted but the deposit didn't clear, the account will erroneously be at zero, when in fact money is still owed. Since the account has already been closed out as paid in full, there will be lost revenue, because collections efforts will not continue. Also, keep in mind that retractions may impact the actual amount that should be posted to a patient's account, so keep this in mind when depositing and posting payments.

✏ Chapter 10 Knowledge Check

Deposit Management and Internal Controls

Question #1:

True or False?   EHR/PM Software can assist with deposit management.

Question #2:

True or False?   In a small office the same staff person who collects payments should also deposit them into the bank

Question #3

True or False? Posting payments prior to deposit assists with expediting of successfully and accurately closing out accounts.

Answers:
Q1: True,
Q2: False,
Q3: False

Chapter 11

Payment Posting

Payment posting is an important part of the overall revenue cycle process and should be timely and accurate.

Post all payments received. When EOBs sit for lengthy periods of time, it delays dropping that claim to the secondary payer, to send an invoice out to a patient who has a coinsurance due, or to fight a denial that may potentially be on that EOB.

There are some organizations that match up every code on the EOB when paid for posting payments and there are others that do lump adjustments. The more accurate you document, the more definition your reporting will have. The better your reporting is, the more effectively you can strategically plan for the future of your organization.

> **Fee Schedule:** A fee schedule is a complete listing of fees used by a payer to reimburse providers and suppliers.

Master Fee Schedules (also known as Charge Masters)

Master fee schedules often have higher amounts than contractually negotiated amounts. This is by design, so a practice captures the allowable rate. A practice may negotiate the reimbursement for CPT 99213 at $65 with one company and $75 with another. The charges, however, should not vary by payer. So, a billed charge of $65 will only be paid out at $65, even if that payer has a $75 allowable charge. Payers will not reimburse greater than the amount billed. Payers normally reimburse the lesser of the charges or the allowable.

For this reason, the master fee schedule should reflect a slightly higher amount than the maximum the practice anticipates receiving from any payer in their network. Organizations have different methodologies for creating their master fee schedule but generally use an overall increase of a federal or state fee schedule. For example, some practices bill 120% of Medicare rates, whereas others feel 150% of Medicaid rates are more appropriate.

To begin assessing your master fee schedule, first pull a report of your top 25-50 most frequently billed CPT® codes and the reimbursement rates. Make sure the codes are current. If you discover frequently billed codes that are also frequently denied, then perform additional coding assessments prior to moving forward.

Identify whether there were any codes reimbursed for the exact amount billed. This is an indication that your fee schedule is too low. Likewise, assess whether there are any codes paid for half of the amount billed. This is an indication that either your fee schedule is too high or that you need to consider renegotiation of your payer contracts.

The practice expense, also referred to as overhead or costs of care, should be appropriately calculated when conducting rate setting. Many practices that use Medicare as a benchmark for rate setting also use it as an indicator for overhead costs of care. It's very unlikely that a practice's overhead costs would be equal to the Medicare set rates. Ensure that a commercial payer's standard fee schedule reimburses at a level that covers overhead expenses. Review the master fee schedule at least once a year. Table 11.1 shows a sample fee schedule.

SHOUT OUT GUY

Keep in mind that modifiers and POS codes can affect reimbursement. For example, if you bill a bilateral procedure, there is no need to double the charge amount. The modifier -50 indicates bilateral performance.

Table 11.1 Sample Fee Schedule

CPT Code	Description	Charge Amount 150% of Medicare	Payer #1 Medicare	Payer #2 Medicaid	Payer #3 AEIOU Health	Payer#4 Blue Horse & Green Leaves	Payer#5 Blue Horse & Green Leaves	Payer#6 Cryptic Insurance	Payer#7 Unicorn
99211	Est. Pt. Level 1 Problem Focused	$34.80	$23.20	$19.82	$25.00	$22.00	$24.00	$35.00	$30.00
99212	Est. Pt.- Level 2 Ext. Problem Focused	$75.15	$50.10	$43.03	$55.00	$40.00	$44.00	$55.00	$47.00
99213	Est. Pt.-Level 3 Detailed	$124.94	$83.29	$71.91	$90.00	$85.00	$87.00	$95.00	$88.00
99214	Est. Pt.-Level 4 Comp./mod. complex	$185.44	$122.29	$105.75	$130.00	$124.00	$126.00	$135.00	$125.00
99215	Est. Pt.-Level 5 Comp./high complex	$246.56	$164.37	$142.34	$175.00	$165.00	$168.00	$188.00	$174.00

*The rates listed are fictitious and do not represent any insurance reimbursements.

Let's do a quick analysis of the above sample fee schedule data:

- This practice chose to use 150% of the current year's Medicare fee schedule to develop their charge amounts.
- Quite often, Medicaid is one of the practice's lowest paying insurance. In this instance, Payer #4 is reimbursing $3.03 less than Medicaid for the 99212. Review this area further.
- Overall it appears that Cryptic Insurance is the highest reimbursing payer, followed by Unicorn Insurance and AEIOU Health. This information is important, as we would want to prioritize the lowest paying insurer for fee schedule and rate negotiations. In this example, Blue Horse & Green Leaves Insurance is the lowest paying.

Sliding or Self-Pay Fee Schedules

Practices commonly maintain a separate fee schedule on a sliding-scale for patients who do not have insurance. These fee schedules are referred to as sliding or self-pay. Though the terms are used interchangeably, they have different meanings. Self-pay simply indicates the patient is solely responsible for payment. It does not directly indicate that any reduction in payment. Sliding schedules indicate that the patient's income or another financial metric is used as a benchmark to determine what the patient can afford to pay for services.

The master fee schedule includes a buffer to capture allowable amounts. For self-pay patients, this does not apply; therefore, billing a lower rate that is more reflective of cost is appropriate. A good place to start is with a review of the average allowable rate by procedure. Use that as the basis of the self-pay fee schedule.

Be cautious when using a sliding-fee scale. Providers who participate with Medicare are not permitted to reduce or waive payments for covered services for Medicare beneficiaries. Most commercial plans include similar requirements in their provider contracts and/or participation guidelines.

> SHOUT OUT GUY
>
> Do not generate multiple master fee schedules for providers in the same practice unless they have differing specialties or another clearly identifiable reason for the difference.

Explanation of Benefits (EOBs) and Electronic Remittance Advice (ERAs)

These two documents provide practices with the information needed to either post payments manually or to confirm electronically posted payments. The goals of the EOB and ERA are to provide all information needed to reconcile any discrepancies between charges billed and payments received. Figure 11.1 shows an example of an EOB. Individuals may use these terms interchangeably, because the ERA is simply an electronic version of an EOB.

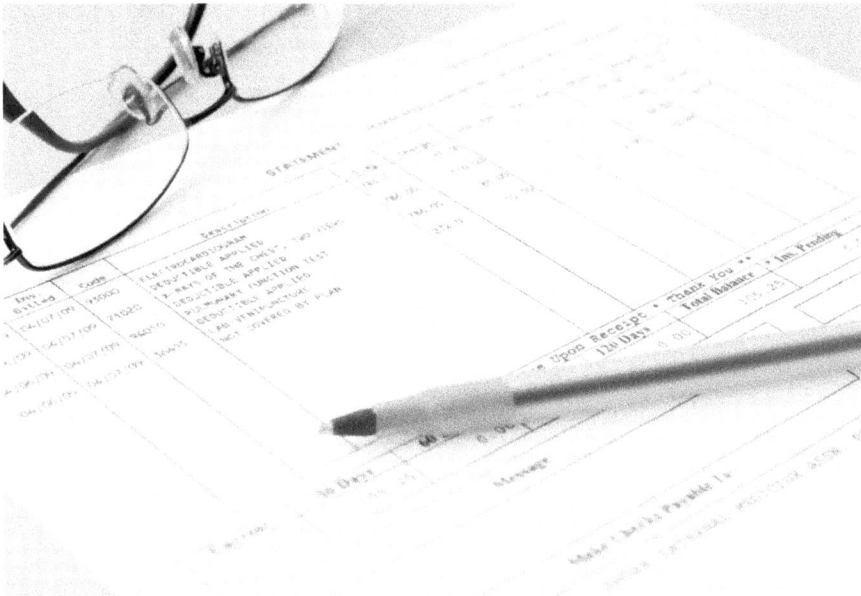

Figure 11.1   An Explanation of Benefits

In addition to amounts paid, other information is available on the EOB or ERA, including contractual adjustments, patient responsibilities, sequestration amounts, quality program bonuses/penalties, and denials of payment.[1] There will be an associated claim adjustment reason code (CARC) for all adjustments that identify why the reduction was made. For some CARCs, there will also be remittance advice remark codes (RARC). For more information, refer to http://www.wpc-edi.com/reference/.

For the rest of this section, we will refer to two sample EOBs shown as Figures 11.2 and 11.3:

Cutten Mend Health Insurance
Explanation of Benefits

Patient Provider	DOS	Proc	Mod	Billed	Allowed	Pt. Resp	Paid	Remark
John Doe Dr. Smitha	1/1/2021	99213		100.00	00	00	00	PR-2, PR-3 CO45
	1/1/2021	96372	25	25.00	00	00	00	PR-2 C)-45
			Total	125.00	00	00	00	

Remark Codes
PR-2 Patient Coinsurance
PR-3 Patient Copay
CO-45 Charge exceeds maximum Allowable

Payment : Check
Tracking# : 123456
Date : 1/31//2021

Figure 11.2   Sample EOB #1

Cutten Mend Health Insurance
Explanation of Benefits

Patient Provider	DOS	Proc	Mod	Billed	Allowed	Pt. Resp	Paid	Remark
John Doe Dr. Smitha	1/1/2021	99213		100.00	00	00	00	PR-2, PR-3 CO45
	1/1/2021	96372	25	25.00	00	00	00	PR-2 C)-45
			Total	125.00	00	00	00	

Remark Codes
PR-2 Patient Coinsurance
PR-3 Patient Copay
CO-45 Charge exceeds maximum Allowable

Payment : Check
Tracking# : 123456
Date : 1/31//2021

Figure 11.3   Sample EOB #2

Contractual Adjustments

Contractual adjustments are amounts deducted from the total payment based on your contractual agreement with the payer. As described above, the practice's master fee schedule will reflect rates that are higher than negotiated amounts. If the practice charges $100 for CPT 99213 but have negotiated a reimbursement of $80, then $20 will be subtracted as a contractual adjustment. An example of this sort of adjustment is shown in Figure 11.2.

Some EOBs will have a column for adjustment amounts, but others will not. It is important to review EOBs closely. There isn't a separate column for the $20 contractual adjustment in Figure 11.2; however, there is a CARC indicating that an adjustment occurred: CO-45, charge exceed maximum allowable.

CARCs versus RARCs

Usually, CARCs are listed by procedure code line. Some CARCs will require additional explanation. For example, CO-226 means "Information requested from the Billing/Rendering Provider was not provided or not provided timely or was insufficient/incomplete." This CARC requires the attachment of at least one RARC. [2]

RARCs provide more information regarding the adjusted amount. Using the example above with CARC CO-226, the attached RARC might be M26, which is defined as:

> The information furnished does not substantiate the need for this level of service. If you have collected any amount from the patient for this level of service/any amount that exceeds the limiting charge for the less extensive service, the law requires you to refund that amount to the patient within 30 days of receiving this notice.

These codes are updated regularly, so we encourage the use of an electronic reference guide if your clearinghouse or PM system doesn't automatically convert this information for you.

When a payer fails to pay in a timely manner, the practice may be due interest on top of the allowed amount. Use adjustment code CO-225 to document interest payments received from insurance companies. Though this may not occur often, you do need a mechanism to post and track the interest payment and to ensure the total amount posted in your practice management systems matches the total payment received. To trend interest payments, run a report of CO-225 by financial class to identify late payment trends. Details about late payments can be found in your payer contracts and your state insurance commissioner's office.

When a payer fails to pay in a timely manner, the practice may be due interest on top of the allowed amount. Use adjustment code CO-225 to document interest payments received from insurance companies. Though this may not occur often, you do need a mechanism to post and track the interest payment and to ensure the total amount posted in your practice management systems matches the total payment received. To trend interest payments, run a report of CO-225 by financial class to identify late payment trends. Details about late payments can be found in your payer contracts and your state insurance commissioner's office.

Patient Responsibilities

Patients have contractual obligations to their insurance company. The primary obligations you will see noted on EOBs will be copays, deductibles, and coinsurance amounts due. (See Chapter 5 for more description of these terms.)

> SHOUT OUT GUY Patients have contractual obligations to their insurance company. The primary obligations you will see noted on EOBs will be copays, deductibles, and coinsurance amounts due. (See Chapter 5 for more description of these terms.)

Refer again Figure 11.2. As with contractual adjustments, CARCs identify the reasoning behind the patient responsibilities. In the CARCs, you can see that the patient had a copay due and a coinsurance due.

Therefore, these amounts weren't in the total payment as it is now the responsibility of the practice to collect from the patient.

If the patient has additional insurance (secondary, tertiary, etc.) their copays may not be their responsibility. Verify claim submission to all active and appropriate insurance payers prior to invoicing the patient. (For more information on multiple insurance and coordination of benefits, refer to Chapter 6.)

Sequestration

Unfortunately, for the foreseeable future, sequestration continues to apply to federal payment programs. This means that, at least through 2027, there is a federal reduction of 2% as a federal cost savings measure.

Monitor commercial agreements closely, as there have been instances of commercial plan alignment to the sequestration reduction. As seen in Figure 11.3, sequestration reductions will come with CARC 253. Table 11.2 provides a sequestration example. According to the Congressional Budget Office (CBO), "Sequestration refers to automatic spending cuts that occur through the withdrawal of funding for certain (but not all) government programs."[3]

Providers should check the CBO website at least annually to determine whether a sequestration will be required at https://www.cbo.gov/taxonomy/term/33/latest. [4]

Table 11.2	American College of Physicians - Medicare Part B Sequestration Payment Sample	
	Allowed amount	$100.00
	Beneficiary coinsurance	($100 x 20%) = $20
	Payment to physician	($100 x 80%) - 2% = $78.40

https://www.ACP.com/practice resources

Sustainable Growth Rate (SGR)

Healthcare spending has long been an expense that requires oversight and cost-control. The SGR was included in the Balanced Budget Act of 1997 to control physician payments within the Medicare program by tying annual increased Medicare Physician Fee Schedule (MPFS) spending to national economic growth.

The 2015 Medicare Access and CHIP Reauthorization Act (MACRA) law replaced the flawed SGR formula while keeping in place the MPFS. MACRA consolidated previous quality programs, like PQRS and Meaningful Use, into the Quality Payment Program (QPP).

Quality Program Bonuses/Penalties

Quality programs include methodologies for assessing bonuses and penalties to providers based upon specific performance metrics. These bonuses and penalties appear on EOBs with corresponding claim adjustment reason codes.

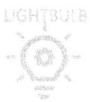

> LIGHTBULB Billing managers: do not accept quality program adjustments at face value without verification. Confirm with management that the reduction/increase is appropriate. Practice managers: keep your billing manager/department updated on quality program performance outcomes and the impact, if any, that performance will have on upcoming reimbursements.

The dream of physicians is to offer patients a care plan that reaches all members of the care team and places the patient's priorities and needs first. Clinically Integrated Networks and Accountable Care Organizations allow for that communication and coordination to occur. Reorganizing the care process around the patient's priorities should be the new standard. For the private practicing physician, the returns can be realized in streamlined workflows, better adherence to best practices, better patient satisfaction, and wellness.[5]

Aimee Yu, MD, MBA

Accountable Care Organizations (ACOs) are groups of doctors, hospitals, and other health care providers who come together voluntarily to give coordinated high-quality care to their Medicare patients. Many practices see value in participating in an ACO. One benefit is coordinated and integrated care. ACO members also benefit from mutually agreed upon quality measures, which in turns allows for shared savings and the potential for higher rates of reimbursement. Additionally, ACO participants can take advantage of Group Purchasing Organizations that allow for volume-based discounts on supplies and services. The participants can also leverage the larger group in payer reimbursement negotiations.

Denials of Payment

As discussed earlier, there are many reasons for payment denials, if the full claims preparation process occurred, then the denial is likely due to something outside of your control. For example, coverage lapses that are gaps in a patient's insurance/benefit coverage. These can occur for many reasons and occasionally occur retroactively. Another common denial reason is "information required from patient." Sometimes an insurance company requires additional demographic, historical, or socio-economic information and will withhold benefit payments as incentive for the patient to respond.

If the claims preparation process did not occur, then the denial may have internal causes like a failure to include a required referral or authorization, an incorrect supervising/rendering provider, or missing documentation for a visit. Other internal denials include code mismatches, which will be things like POS to CPT® mismatches, diagnosis to CPT® mismatches, and modifier to CPT® mismatches.

223

Examples of code mismatches include billing a hospital CPT® code with a private practice POS code, billing an appendectomy with the diagnosis of diabetes as opposed to appendicitis, and using an excluded modifier for a CPT®. To avoid these mishaps, it is imperative that a current CPT® and ICD book be utilized.

Denials look somewhat like the record for Jane Doe in Figure 11.3. The total charges are $100, and the payments are listed as $0. The CARC identifies the reason for the payment denial. In this case, Jane's appointment occurred before her coverage began. For additional information about CARCs and RARCs refer to Chapter 12.

SHOUT OUT GUY Occasionally, patients fail to pay insurance premiums and the insurer cancels retroactively. In these situations, it is appropriate to bill the patient. In the situation described above, this could have been identified before the patient's appointment occurred. (For more information on proper review of eligibility and verifications, refer to Chapter 4.)

EOB/Remittance Management

Management of remittances and EOBs relies upon a few easy tasks like confirming the receipt of payment for every EOB/ERA received and an EOB/ERA for every payment received. Regularly reviewing outstanding A/R to identify any missing remittances and having a process for retention as well as a process for retrieval for review when needed are also excellent ways to help strategically manage remittances.

Write-Offs versus Contractual Adjustments

Some people use these terms interchangeably, but they are *not* the same thing. Contractual adjustments, as outlined above, are required adjustments based upon provider or facility participations agreements. Write-offs are amounts that were electively adjusted-off.

Write-off reasons include:

Missed timely filing windows. Each insurer allows a window of time to appeal denials. They will deny claims appealed outside of this window and will prohibit patient billing.

Failure to obtain prior authorization. Each insurer has a list of procedures, services, and medications which require pre-approval or *prior authorization*. Failure to obtain these approvals is a violation of the provider's participation agreement with the insurer. The insurer will deny claims that lack required authorizations and will often prohibit patient billing.

Missing referrals. Some insurers/plans require referrals from the primary care physician. Failure to obtain these referrals is a violation of the provider's participation agreement with the insurer. The insurer will deny claims that lack required referrals and prohibit patient billing.

Missing ABN. The advance beneficiary notice (ABN) is a form stating the patient is aware they will have a financial responsibility for a future service. This is a requirement when future services not covered and the patient elects to continue regardless. (For more information, see Chapter 4 and Chapter 6.) The insurer will deny claims that lack required ABNs and will prohibit patient billing.

Contractual Adjustments = Expected Decrease in Payment
Write-Offs = Typically Preventable Losses

Management should review the write-offs report at least monthly to identify trends and potential problem areas. Financial hardships and demise are examples of write-off reasons. To report individually, it's important to code write-offs into separate categories.

If the write-offs fall into preventable areas, then re-education of staff must occur. You will want to create and implement stricter measures if write-offs occur often.

Virtual Credit Card Payments

Virtual credit card (VCC) payments are a newer method of reimbursement. The practice will receive VCCs either via fax, mail, or EHR portal. The VCC will include remittance information along with credit card processing information for the total EOB payment amount due.

> SHOUT OUT GUY Accepting VCC payments is a choice not a requirement; to change payment types, contact the number on the VCC payment form and request payment via EFT or check. It takes just as long to mail a check as it does to have a VCC slip mailed, and a check won't cost you any credit card transaction fees.
>
> The fees associated with accepting VCC payments are deducted from the contracted allowable amount that would have been paid to the practice for services. This means the practice will be paid less per beneficiary every time a VCC is accepted as a form of payment.

Be wary of VCC payments. Merchant service providers (see Chapter 6) charge fees to run credit card payments. The fees are generally a percentage of the total amount processed and can be as much as 5-8%. This means, by accepting virtual payments, you will be paying a fee to receive money that is already due to you. In the state of Maryland, both authors supported the Maryland MGMA's Government Affairs committee in changing legislation to help protect practices against virtual payment fees. We continue to encourage state associations and their members to engage in local legislation that protects and supports your practice. Contact your local MGMA for information on how to get involved.

✎ Chapter 11 Knowledge Check

Payment Posting

Question #1:
Explain how a contractual adjustment is different from an allowed amount.

Question #2:
Are Medicare products the only payers impacted by sequestration adjustments?

Question #3:
What is the difference between an EOB and an ERA?

Question #4:
Master fee schedules often have _____ amounts than contractually negotiated amounts.

Question #5:
Sequestration is a federal reduction of _____ as a federal cost savings measure

Question #6:
It is common for practices to maintain a separate fee schedule on a sliding-scale for patients who do not have insurance. These are often called the _____ or _____ fee schedules

---

Answers:

Q1: Contractual adjustments are amounts deducted from the total payment based on your contractual agreement with the payer. The allowed amount is the contracted amount for the provided service(s).

Q2: No. Some payer contracts have included alignment in the language.

Q3: EOB is short for Explanation of Benefits. ERA is short for Electronic Remittance Advice. These terms can be used interchangeably as ERA is the electronic version of an EOB.

Q4: higher

Q5: 2%

Q6: sliding or self-pay

Endnotes

1. https://www.cms.gov/Outreach-and-Education/Medicare-Learning-Network-MLN/MLNProducts/Downloads/Remit-Advice-Overview-Fact-Sheet-ICN908325.pdf

2. http://www.wpc-edi.com/reference/

3. https://www.cbo.gov/topics/budget/sequestration

4. https://www.cbo.gov/taxonomy/term/33/latest

5. Book quote provide by: *Aimee Yu, MD, MBA*

Chapter 12

Denial Management

Additional steps in the RCM are required as the medical community shifts from the FFS model to the pay-for-performance (P4P) model, also referred to as the value-based payment model. This transition comes with additional billing requirements and reviews to determine whether all claims were processed correctly and paid. Today, most practices have moved to receiving ERAs in lieu of paper EOBs. ERAs allow staff to manage, review, and post electronically.

Using your PM software and having access to your practice's clearinghouse are critical components for supervision and growth. Prior to setting up electronic remittances, notify insurance companies of the intention to accept ERAs. This change will allow your team to post payments quicker or to set your practice management system up for auto-posting.

Upon receiving the ERA, confirm receipt of payment through either a paper check or an EFT. EFTs are the fastest method of reimbursement for the organization and, unlike VCCs, do not come with additional fees to process into your bank account. When the payment has been confirmed, review the payments, adjustments, and remarks for each patient. If you followed the recommendation to populate the allowable amounts for each insurance payer into your PM system, then the process for review will be expedient. Regardless of the method you use, it is vital that you confirm payments are accurate, review non-payments, and look for denial trends.

Denials and non-payments can significantly impact the revenue cycle in both FFS and P4P models, so proactive preventive management of denials is vital.

SHOUT OUT GUY Payer correspondence is essential to review. Whether received through the mail, via payer portal, or through other electronic means, payers communicate critical information through their correspondence to your organization. Payer correspondence will identify policy changes, claim denials, payment issues, fee schedule changes, audits, and more. Payers will also notify you of an intent to terminate or to make other changes to your contract through correspondence.

Have a set process for how the practice handles payer correspondence and make sure to reduce the number of people involved to as few as possible. Ideally, payer correspondence should go directly to billing for processing prior to any other department reviewing.

Proactive, Preventive Approach

The best method for management of denials is to prevent them from occurring in the first place. This means taking a proactive approach. Anticipate potential denial issues and create internal controls to prevent them. Figure 12.1 shows a few examples of opportunities to prevent denials:

The above graphic contains just a handful of examples. To truly optimize your denial prevention methods, critically review your workflows and business processes. Do they prevent opportunities for denials? If not, what processes could you implement to help ensure denial prevention?

If you are already receiving denials, think about how they occur and implement processes to head them off.

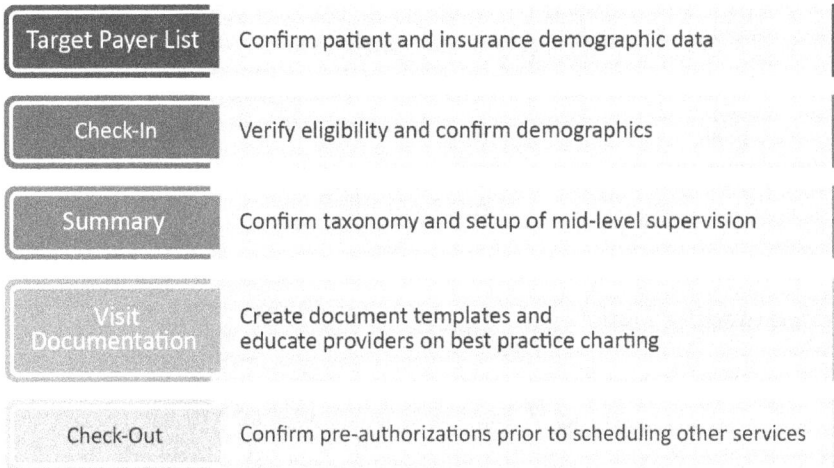

Target Payer List	Confirm patient and insurance demographic data
Check-In	Verify eligibility and confirm demographics
Summary	Confirm taxonomy and setup of mid-level supervision
Visit Documentation	Create document templates and educate providers on best practice charting
Check-Out	Confirm pre-authorizations prior to scheduling other services

Figure 12.1   Opportunities to prevent denials

Non-Payment

A non-payment is not necessarily a denial of payment, and it's important to understand the difference between the two terms. A non-payment is a claim that has been adjudicated but unpaid. Sometimes this simply means the insurance company requires additional information prior to full adjudication of that claim. The practice then has an opportunity to provide the necessary information to ensure receipt of payment. For example, an insurance company may opt not to pay for a service because there is a question of whether service was medically necessary to perform. In this situation, in order to move from a non-payment to a payment status, the practice would need to justify the medical necessity for the unpaid service period.

To confirm medical necessity with the insurance payer, the practice will need to send documentation of services rendered and any related or corroborating documents. These documents, once received by the payer, will be reviewed, and the claim will be reconsidered.

231

Denial of Payment

A denial of payment means the claim was fully adjudicated and payment was determined to be unwarranted. As mentioned earlier, denial reasons will vary. Some claims are denied because they contain services that cannot be billed together, others are denied because an authorization was not submitted with the claim, and some claims are denied because the records received and reviewed were insufficient. Some of the reasons given for denying claims can and should be appealed.

Understanding Denials

In the previous chapter, we reviewed Claim Adjustment Reason Codes (CARCs) and Remittance Advice Remark Codes (RARCs). These codes act as a legend to explain the impetus behind the insurer's denial of payment.

Insurance remittances will either contain descriptions for these codes on each page, list them on the final page, or provide information on where to find descriptions online. One such resource is the reference section of the Washington Publishing Company at http://www.wpc-edi.com/reference/. Here you will find a list of over 200 CARCs and many more RARCs.

COMPUTER Finding an online resource is very helpful for your staff, as these codes are updated three times a year. Also, on electronic resources your team can take advantage of the find or search option on a webpage to quickly locate the codes and descriptions they are seeking out. On a Microsoft Windows-based computer, you can open the search bar by pressing CTRL+F, on an Apple Mac-based computer, press COMMAND+F.

Common CARCs & RARCs

A breakout of some common CARCs[1] and RARCs[2] are listed in Table 12.1, with key points of reference:

Table 12.1 Some Common CARCs

CARC	Description
PR-1	Deductible amount
CO-50	These are non-covered services because this is not deemed a medical necessity by the payer.
CO-96	Non-covered charge(s)
CO-18	Duplicate claim/service
CO-97	The benefit for this service is included in the payment or allowance for another service or procedure that has already been adjudicated.
CO-B12	Services not documented in patient's medical records
CO-49	This is a non-covered service because it is a routine/preventive exam, or a diagnostic/screening procedure done in conjunction with a routine/preventive exam

Note that the first two CARCs begin with different pre-fixes, PR and CO these represent Claim Adjustment Group Codes.:

CO - Contractual Obligations

OA - Other Adjustments

PI - Payer Initiated Reductions

PR - Patient Responsibility

RARCs will not be provided for all CARCs. They are used to convey supplemental or informational messages; the latter will be prefaced with Alert. It is easy to identify RARCs on ERAs and EOBs because they will begin with the letter M or the letter N. A few RARCs have been listed in Table 12.2 as an example.

Table 12.2 Some Common RARCs	
RARC	**Description**
M15	Separately billed services/tests have been bundled as they are considered components of the same procedure. Separate payment is not allowed.
M53	Missing/incomplete/invalid days or units of service.
N199	Additional payment/recoupment approved based on payer-initiated review/audit.

Note that the above RARCs are providing additional insight into denials that help guide you in how to potentially recoup payment. RARCs will not be listed without a CARC. For example, you may see CO-B12 or PI-B12 on a claim coupled with N199. These two codes together let you know there was a payer-initiated review/audit and that a payment originally made was rescinded due to the services not being documented in the patient's medical record.

Many of the CARCs and RARCs that exist can be prevented through proper management, staff education, and training. Table 12.3 provides several examples of denials that could easily be preventively managed:

Table 12.3   Preventable Denials

CARC	Description	Resolution
96	Non-covered charges.	Prior to performing or billing a service, ensure that the service is covered under Medicare. Please refer to the CMS Internet-Only Manual, 100-02, Chapter 16.[3]
49	Payment is denied when performed/ billed by this type of provider.	Ensure that provider setup in the PM system includes alignment of taxonomy to specialty.

97	The benefit for this service is included in the payment or allowance for another service or procedure that has already been adjudicated.	Verify prior to service being rendered whether the service being billed is bundled into payment for another service or considered part of a global surgical package, or part of a more comprehensive service already billed.
50	These are non-covered services because this is not deemed a medical necessity by the payer.	Follow Medicare guidelines, national and local coverage determinations for the service billed. Education of Medicare changes will assist in this process. When applicable, utilize ABNs.[4]
B7	This provider was not covered by Medicare when the patient received this service	This provider was not certified/eligible to be paid for this procedure/service on this date of service. Confirm credentialing status. Acceptance into the Medicare Part B program will allow additional revenue that is not reimbursed by Medicare Part A. An example would be for nebulizer treatments. The treatment and drug charges would be reimbursed under Part B services, otherwise the service is denied by Part A.[5]

In the above listed examples, it's easy to see there are many opportunities to prevent denials: proper system setup, checking eligibility in advance, reviewing local and national coverage determinations, etc.

Even with a proactive approach, there will be times when claims are denied and need to be appealed.

Appealing Denials

To begin the appeal process, first make sure to fully understand the reason for the denial and document necessary recovery steps. The specific protocols will vary by provider. There is standard information that should be included in any denial/payment reconsideration request. These items include, but are not limited to, the patient's full name, the date of service, the provider's full name, the provider's NPI, the provider's TIN, the insurance company's denial reason, and a thorough explanation of the practice's reason for the appeal and reconsideration request of the denial.

When sending an appeal request, be sure to follow each insurance company's guidelines for appeals. Many insurance companies require internal forms or portals to appeal a denial. Denials may be upheld for failure to follow the insurance company's appeals process. The most common reason denials are upheld is not filing within the timely filing window. This means the claim wasn't appealed within the date range required by the payer.

Five Levels of Medicare Appeals

There are five levels in the Medicare Part A and Part B appeals process. The levels are:[6]

- 1st Level of Appeal: Redetermination by a Medicare Administrative Contractor (MAC)[7]
- 2nd Level of Appeal: Reconsideration by a Qualified Independent Contractor (QIC)
- 3rd Level of Appeal: Decision by the Office of Medicare Hearings and Appeals (OMHA)
- 4th Level of Appeal: Review by the Medicare Appeals Council
- 5th Level of Appeal: Judicial Review in Federal District Court

For more information on the Medicare Appeal process, navigate to: https://www.cms.gov/Medicare/Appeals-and-Grievances/OrgMedFFS Appeals/index.html.

Higher Level Appeals

State insurance commissioners are responsible for oversight of insurance companies. Once a practice has exhausted the insurance company's internal appeals process, it is highly recommended that they move on to requesting support from the state insurance administration. Notably, the state insurance commission will not overturn denials where the organization failed to comply with their contractual obligations. Prior to seeking support from an insurance commissioner, be sure that you have followed the health plan's outlines related to claim submissions, clean claims, and any contract specifications that your practice has signed within your Participation Agreement. Review your denial, appeal, provider agreement, and payer policy manual prior to reaching out to the state insurance commissioner. In the event a practice has not followed these guidelines, the insurance administration will not be able to intervene.

The state insurance commissioners ensure that each insurance company follows the guidelines set by that state legislature in coordination with the state's insurance administration. For more information, navigate to the National Association of Insurance Commissioners at https://www.naic.org/state_web_map.htm; at this site you can pull up your state representative and their contact information.

If an insurance company did not follow state law when denying a medical service, then the insurance administration agency could be of help. Please note that the insurance administration agency cannot get involved in self-funded, federally funded, or state-funded denials. This includes denials from Medicare and Medicaid among other payers.

The federal plans would include plans such as Federal Blue Cross Blue Shield, Tricare,

And any other federally funded health plan that is exempt from oversight from the insurance administration.

Timely Filing

As you consider denial management and revenue cycle improvements, also take into consideration timely filing limits. Each insurance company has their own guidelines for the time allowed for a provider to submit a claim. This amount of time begins on the date of service.

The chart presented in Table 12.4 is an example of the type of timely filing chart you should maintain. Please review your group and provider agreements with the payer to confirm actual timelines.

Table 12.4   Example Timely Filing Chart

Payer	Referral Required	Timely Filing	Timely Appeals
AETNA HMO	YES	6 MONTHS	3 MONTHS
AETNA PPO	NO	6 MONTHS	3 MONTHS
AETNA MEDCR SUPP.	NO	15 MONTHS	120 DAYS AFTER CLAIM PAID
BCBS PPO	NO	1 YEAR	6 MONTHS
BCBS FED	NO	1 YEAR	6 MONTHS
BCBS HMO'S (Not all require referrals; some have Open Access)	HMO/ REF REQ	1 YEAR	6 MONTHS
CIGNA PPO	NO	6 MONTHS	6 MONTHS
HUMANA	NO	6 MONTHS	6 MONTHS
KAISER	YES		
UHC	YES	6 MONTHS	3 MONTHS
TRICARE PRIME	YES	1 YEAR	6 MONTHS

In the event that a claim is submitted past the timely filing limits for an insurance company, it is very unlikely that claim will be paid. Review participation agreements and document the timely limits accordingly. Insurance payers and insurance commissioners will support timely filing denial decisions.

Once you've created a timely filing matrix, make it available to front office and billing staff alike. This payer participation list could also include any requirements for referrals or prior authorizations based on your practice's specialty.

Trending Denials

Trending denials is an important diagnosis tool when reviewing the overall revenue cycle. A great way to trend denials would be based on CPT code, insurance company, provider, and denial reason. Trending denials using these factors will help you identify patterns to address to avoid replicating the same denials. Once denials are trended and identified, it is also important to put processes in place to avoid these denials occurring in the future.

For example, if the practice performs echocardiograms, and receives a denial from a carrier indicating that prior authorization is required, then the prior authorization may be a new or internal protocol change within the carrier's network. In this case, determine the reason for the denial (new service, out-of-network, etc.), and make the appropriate change internally. In most cases, this means obtaining prior authorization in advance of rendering services.

Re-education Reduces Denials

After identifying denial trends, ensure that comprehensive protocols are in place to avoid future denials and communicate these protocols with the necessary staff and providers.

When communicating protocols to staff, it is helpful to give examples of denials as well as the systems created to prevent such denials in the future. Consider sharing this information through staff meetings, morning huddles, practice meetings, email, intra-mail, and through updates to the practice's standard operating procedures manual.

When conducting re-education on denial, prevention, and avoidance, it's a great idea to give anonymized examples of previous denials and to

239

include dollar amounts associated to those denials that will enforce the sense of urgency to comply with new protocols. It is not unusual for the denial reasons to be related to issues at check-in. Accurate registration and updates to patient demographics are critical.

It is ideal to have an internal scrubbing process as outlined in Chapter 9. Review this claim's scrubbing process as part of the re-education process.

Recoupments, Retractions, and Takebacks

Sometimes an insurance payer will reimburse services initially and then retroactively deny them. This results in a recoupment of payment that may be referred to as a recoupment, retraction, or takeback. This typically happens when an insurance company paid a claim without requesting records and then audited records later down the road or when a patient's insurance retroactively cancels. There are many circumstances under which a payer may retract the initial claim approval and seek a recoupment of payment.

For many payers, the recoupments will be automatically deducted from future reimbursement checks/EFTs; for other payers, your organization will need to issue a check payable to the insurance company to repay them. Recoupments are overpayments and are therefore treated as such.

It is important to document recoupments so they can be appealed if applicable, and so future remittance documents can be properly balanced. Documenting a recoupment on one ERA while the actual funds are removed from a separate transaction can create an imbalance for the payment poster. Make sure to document or otherwise alert staff of initiated recoupments.

To appeal retractions and recoupments, follow standard appeals processes. In some cases, there will not be an opportunity to appeal. Using the example above, if a patient's insurance was retroactively canceled, then you may not be able to get that money back via appeal. You may need to forward the balance to the patient for payment. (Refer to Chapter 14 for more information on *promissory estoppel*).

✏ Chapter 12 Knowledge Check

Denial Management

Question #1:

Petitioning for the reconsideration of a denied claim is called an

_____.

Question #2:

When a payer initially approves a payment and then takes it back this is often referred to as a _____, _____ or a_____

Question #3:

True or False? Insurance verification is a factor in denial management.

Answers:

Q1: Appeals,
Q2: Recoupments, Takebacks or Retractions,
Q3: True

Endnotes

1. http://www.x12.org/codes/claim-adjustment-reason-codes/

2. http://www.wpc-edi.com/reference/codelists/healthcare/remittance-advice-remark-codes/

3. https://www.cms.gov/Regulations-and-Guidance/Guidance/Manuals/Downloads/bp102c16.pdf

4. CMS National Coverage Determinations Manual, Pub. 100-03: https://www.cms.gov/Regulations-and-Guidance/Guidance/Manuals/Internet-Only-Manuals-IOMs-Items/CMS014961.html?DLPage=1&DLSort=0&DLSortDir=ascending

5. www.cms.gov/Medicare/Medicare-Fee-for-Service payment/PhysicianFeeSched/index.html

6. https://www.cms.gov/Medicare/Appeals-and-Grievances/OrgMedFFSAppeals/index.html

7. https://www.cms.gov/Medicare/Appeals-and-Grievances/OrgMedFFSAppeals/index.html

Chapter 13

Insurance A/R Follow-Up

Insurance A/R is one of the most important revenue indicators in a medical practice. Attention to insurance A/R is vital to the financial health of a medical practice. Devote dedicated time and resources to this very important responsibility. Continued professional development and education of resources assigned to insurance A/R is critical to keeping staff aware of reimbursement changes and improve collections techniques.

Remaining current on reimbursement and guideline changes is a key factor to timely collections and the ability to increase revenue based on the ever-changing updates. Medicare and other insurance companies make updates to payment policies annually. Education and adaptability are essential to maximizing potential revenue.

Your practice's EHR/PM software support is essential to the insurance A/R follow-up process, so understanding the features available in the software during software selection is key. Review of A/R reports, tracking features, notification systems, and claim submissions are all important. If you are leaving one software and transitioning to another, consider determining the data and format that your old software can provide, along with the data and format that the new software is able to accept. Identify costs associated to data extraction (from old software) and data upload (to new software). Ensure that all data is in a secure HIPAA-compliant format. Make sure that the timing of data transition fits the practices needs. For more information on switching EHRs and considerations during transition, refer to the ONC's publication on transition issues at: https://www.healthit.gov/sites/default/files/playbook/pdf/ehr-contract-guide-chapter-9.pdf.

> COMPUTER Speak with your EHR representative to discuss integration methods, close open ports, and otherwise ensure HIPAA compliance.

Proactively review and create an internal action plan to include annual reimbursement changes and fee schedules. Reimbursement for services rendered is a complex network of obstacles from government mandates to intricate rules by individual payers that Is going to be successfully tackled through teamwork, investigation, streamlining processes, and staying aware of reimbursement guidelines.

To optimize staff's success, ensure that appropriate personnel have necessary access to data and software permissions. Staff who are responsible for payment posting, but who are not privy to deposit information, will have a tough time performing these functions and being able to reconcile. Staff who are responsible for A/R follow up will not be able to manage claims edits and denials unless they are privy to the claim submission process. Intake and registration staff who are unaware of missing patient information, such as insurance cards, listing of primary care physician on insurance cards for PCP services, will not be as effective in denial prevention during the registration process.

Aging A/R

Ideally, we would prevent aging balances by having stellar prevention processes. When claims are unpaid and aging, address them with strategy and a sense of urgency. As charges increase, so should collections. Internal practice factors that can impact charges include missed appointments, provider productivity decrease, and practice availability decrease. Rule out these factors and begin looking for other issues within the revenue cycle.

An industry best practice is to manage insurance A/R report generation. A few areas of concentration when working from an insurance A/R unpaid aging report include high dollar amounts, aging over 45 days, coding discrepancies, registration errors, payer reimbursement rules, possible duplicate claims, and credentialing issues.

The goal is to minimize aging A/R by ensuring claims are *clean* when submitted. Insurance A/R is specifically the amount owed to a provider by an insurance company for covered services, as opposed to other parties who owe the practice money.

As owed amounts age, they are divided into periods, as shown in Figure 13.1:

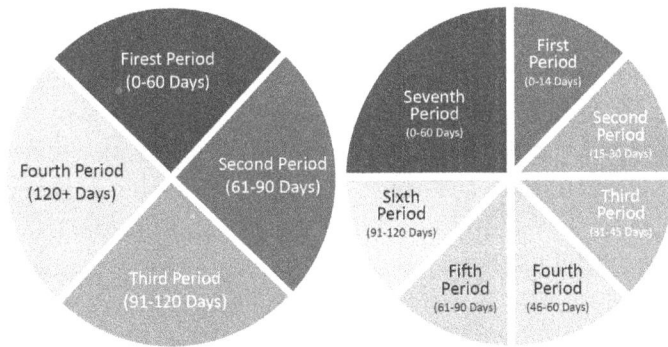

Figure 13.1   Traditional Claim Lifecycle Compared
to Recommended Claim Lifecycle

Reviewing the above graphic, you can see that the goal is to get more periods of review in the first 90 days. In a traditional review model, there would be two periods of review in the first 90 days of the claim. In our recommended model, there are five periods of review in the first 90 days.

The first 90 days are critical to timely filing, coordination of benefits corrections, and more. In the table below, we've outlined the differences between the first two review periods of each model. By the end of the second period in the recommended model, the claim is only 30 days old and major delays have already been identified and mitigated.

Insurance Aging Review Cycle

In order to begin working A/R in the recommended bracket, you'll want to be aware of each payer's payment guidelines. For example, Medicare usually pays within 7-14 days and commercial payers may pay within 30 days. Know your insurance payment schedules to determine when it's time to start following up on a claim. Also, check your state's guidelines on insurance company payment notification timelines to be sure that payers are following requirements for payment status notification. Guidelines regarding timelines for reimbursement notification and methods for which a payer will notify a practice related to specific claims should also be in your payer participation agreement.

If you do elect to follow a traditional model, keep in mind that the third aging bucket will include claims that are already greater than three months old. Hopefully claims within this aging bucket have already been addressed and are awaiting a response or resolution from a payer. If a practice has not addressed claims aging in this bucket, a major error has occurred in the A/R follow up or claim submission process. Try not to allow claims to get to this point without any intervention. If a claim is within this bucket, there is also a danger that the claim may not have been received by the payer. In this case, be sure to refer to payer timely filing and timely appeals guidelines.

If your practice has a high dollar value of claims aging in this bracket, there could be collections performance issues. Check your state or payer contract for timely appeals deadlines as these impact claims in this aging bracket. The goal is to keep the 120-day aging bracket at 10% or less of total A/R. Aging at 20% or higher of total A/R is a sign that there may be issues to resolve.

Table 13.1 The First Two Periods of Each Model

Traditional	Recommended
0-30 Day Review Period	**0-14 Day Review Period**
Claims that are in this aging bucket (or aging range) reflect the most recent submissions by the provider's practice and are in review for adjudication by the payer. Having the majority of your practice's accounts receivable within the 0-30-day aging bracket is a healthy A/R indicator. It shows that most of the outstanding revenue is recent and pending claims adjudication.	Claims submitted electronically through a clearinghouse are typically adjudicated within 7-14 days from receipt. A practice may utilize an electronic method to check claim status if payment is still outstanding 14 days after submission. If claims information is not yet available, don't fret, give the payer a little more time to complete claims processing.
60-90 Day Review Period	**16-30 Day Review Period**
By this time, the payer has most likely communicated with the practice via the appropriate communication methods (i.e., EOB) or ERA) as to the payment determination. At the time of this aging bucket, the practice should have on file the status of a claim. Ideally, the practice has already begun addressing any non-payment issues. Don't let too much time elapse from the date of claim submission, the date that a payer has informed you of its payment determination, and the date of addressing a denied or unpaid claim. Considering that it can take payers 14-45 days to pay a claim, you don't want your aging A/R to be higher than 60 days. During this time period it is likely that the practice experienced cash flow impact due to delayed payments. Now is a good time to utilize an aging A/R report to help track action already taken and the need for further action or follow up on unpaid claims. As a claim ages, we spend more money and resources collecting on those claims.	If you are like most practices who are tracking the payment cycles and schedules for your top payers, you'll know when to expect incoming deposits and payments. In the event payment doesn't arrive within the expected timeframe for electronically submitted claims, it's time to be proactive and check the claim status. There's no need to wait the full 30-day cycle. This is a great time to begin using the payer's online portal or your clearinghouse to determine the claim status. If there is still no receipt of payment, it's a good idea to check the claim information to ensure there weren't any submission errors such as patient demographic information, patient's benefits, coding, insurance ID numbers, provider ID numbers, or pay-to information.

The Claims Adjudication Process

The claims adjudication process is a set of internal payer rules that a claim must pass through for payment determination. Obtain proof or documentation of timely claims filing during submission so this information is available if needed during timely filing appeal. During this aging timeframe, the practice is awaiting a response from the payer.

If there is no response to a claim's submission the practice should contact the payer to check the status of the claim. Below are several methods for contacting a payer:

Calling the payer

It is a good idea to keep a list of all payer contact information on file for easy access. Staying friendly when speaking with payer representatives is essential to building a rapport (you get more bees with honey than vinegar). If you take the route of calling payers to check claim status, you may speak with the same representatives from time to time. Consider having cordial conversation while getting to the point of your call; they are speaking to the public all day, so they have little patience for long-drawn out discussions.

When calling a payer, consider checking claim status on multiple patients during one call. Make a note of how many patients a payer will allow you to discuss on each call so that you have patient information readily available. Be sure to document each call thoroughly.

Information needed in preparation for a payer phone call:

- Utilize aging A/R report by payer to gather more than one patient with the same insurance.
- Obtain the insurance companies' phone numbers and claims extensions.
- Review the accounts for the patients that you are preparing to call about.

- Gather patient insurance ID number, date of service, claim number or internal control number (ICN) if available, provider number and NPI, denial reason if know, date of service, and charge amount.
- Reference number of call or corrective action to claim(s) in question
- Any documentation from previous phone calls.

On the payer claim status phone call:

- Obtain and document the representative's name.
- Inform the representative that you are calling to check the status of unpaid claims.
- Patient's benefits and eligibility.
- Confirm outcome/status of claim(s).
- Have the representative outline any required corrective action to allow for claim processing.
- Document details of acceptable method of corrective action.

Utilizing the payer's online portal

When utilizing a payer's online portal, securely save pertinent information displayed online regarding the claim adjudication. This information might be critical in the future for an appeal or other reconsideration request. Keep track of payer websites, usernames, and passwords. You'll want to have an access control policy for exiting and terminated staff to avoid access after employment has ended.

Utilizing your clearinghouse

Some clearinghouses have real-time claims adjudication functionality through direct interfaces with payers' databases. Access to this level of detail allows a practice to determine if a claim will be paid, how much will be paid, the amount that needs to be contractually adjusted, errors, claims edits, and patient's responsibility.

> **Clearinghouse:** This is the middleman between the practice and the insurance company. Typically, practices submit claims to the clearinghouse, which performs a review for errors before submitting to the insurance company; this is a critical component for submitting a clean claim.

Table 13.2   Average Occurrence of Pended Claims[1]

Table 1. Reasons for Pended/ Delayed Claims	Percentage of Pended/ Delayed Claims	Average Number of Days Pended/ Delayed
Duplicate Claims Submitted	35%	9
Lack of Necessary Information	12%	11
No Coverage Based on Date of Service	8%	11
Non-covered/Non-network Benefit or Service	7%	5
Coordination of Benefits (COB)	5%	14
Coverage Determination	4%	8
Utilization Review	3%	10
Authorization	3%	20
Invalid Codes Submitted	1%	16
Pre-existing Condition Review	1%	25
Other*	21%	4
Total	100%	9

*Other reasons cited included: Medicare as primary payer, incorrect provider ID, no provider, ineligible provider, possible third-party liability (TPL), provider watch, member alert, multi-surgery manual pricing, and high dollar claims.

Many practices integrate their clearinghouse with their PM software. Doing this allows for a seamless stream of information between the two systems. As mentioned earlier, there is also PM software that has its own built in clearinghouse. Utilizing an integrated clearinghouse allows for claims adjudication data to be available within the patients account. It's also wise to create internal claims edits based on your knowledge of payer reimbursement guidelines. This will stop claims from going out until they are clean.

Documenting Account Notes

After contacting the payer, be sure to document the research from these interactions in the PM software or other internal financial record. It's also helpful to set reminders to follow up on any action items. This documentation should include any action taken toward claims resolution.

Become proactive in addressing unpaid claims that are aging in A/R.

Strategies for Managing Insurance Aging A/R

1. Place appropriate accounts into an automatic follow-up status and have an alert set to prompt for regular assessment.

2. Educate others on the staff on identified denial reasons and patterns that have been resolved. This can be a team effort. Don't keep the information to yourself.

3. Develop account alerts for troublesome accounts to notify anyone who may access that account about its complexities.

Credit balances

To complicate an already complicated A/R, enter in credit balances, the bane of our existence. Credit balances are unsightly signs that something even deeper is wrong with a claim. It indicates there is a significant payment issue requiring review before account reconciliation or zeroing out.

Credit balances prohibit us from seeing true aging balances because they skew our A/R. Addressing credit balances is not only necessary to clean up our A/R, but it is mandatory, as those balances could be monies owed to others who want their money back. For example, returning federal (Medicare or Medicaid) overpayments within 60 days of identification is a statutory requirement.[2]

Identifying Credit Balances/Overpayments

So how do you identify credit balances? There are many ways to do this. The best way is to use your PM system. It is likely a canned report exists that can pull this data for you. It will have a name like "Credit Balances" or "Overpayments." If you don't see one named that, try running a report that shows account balances of <$0.01.

If running reports like this isn't something you're used to, or you don't see a report that meets your needs, then reach out to your PM system vendor for support and guidance. There should be *two* separate reports, one for patient overpayments and one for insurance company overpayments. The process for managing each will be slightly different.

Insurance Credit Balances

Insurance credit balances can take some time to sort through. Below are three common reasons for insurance overpayments:

- Insurance was paid and then subsequently denied.
- Two insurance plans paid as the primary, or other coordination of benefits issues.
- Some party errantly paid the claim twice.

Table 13.3   Sample Insurance Credit Balance Report

Insurance Plan	Plan/Pt ID	Allowable	Receipts	Balance
Big Federal Insurance	001078	200.00	400.00	(200.00)
Brown, Emily	ABC1234	100.00	200.00	(100.00)
Williams, Adam	ABC2356	100.00	200.00	(100.00)
Total Accounts	2	200.00	400.00	(200.00)

Here you can see that Big Federal Insurance is showing a total credit balance of $200.00. Drilling down, we see that it stems from two overpayments of $100.00.

Once you've identified insurance overpayments, you need to dig in further to review the specific patient, date-of-service, and service line that contains the overpayment. Research thoroughly to ensure the credit balance is accurate.[3] During this process, it helps to review all remittances (EOBs or ERAs) received for this claim. Review the remark codes and payments received to identify the error.[4]

For example, the remittance for Big Federal may appear as in Figure 13.2:

Given the remark codes listed, you now know to review other remittances received from other payers for this patient and date-of-service. If it is unclear which payer should be primary, then contact the patient for coordination of benefits.

				Big Federal Care Health Insurance	Explanation of Benefits			
Patient	DOS	Proc	Mod	Billed	Allowed	Pt Resp	Paid	Remark
Brown, Emily	1/1/2021	99213		100.00	0.00	0.00	0.00	22, M43
Williams, Adam	1/1/2021	99213		100.00	0.00	0.00	0.00	22, M43
			TOTAL	200.00	0.00	0.00	0.00	

Remark Codes
22 This care may be covered by another payer per coordination of benefits
M43 Payment for this service previously issued to you or another provider by another carrier/intermediary

Payment: CHECK
Tracking#: 234568
Date: 1/31/2021

Figure 13.2   Example Remittance

Once you review the overpayment, you will either need to refund the insurer, contact the patient to address coordination of benefits issues, or send an appeal or revised claim to the insurer.

Refer to your provider agreements and payer manuals for guidance on dates and timelines.[5] Some manuals will be more specific than others in the information they make available. Federal payments are highly regulated and, as such, much information is available. Many commercial payers follow federal guidelines, but it's important to review each payer contract to ensure practice compliance. Medicare's overpayment guidance is as follows:

There are situations in which you will receive a notice for overpayment collection. This notice is referred to as a demand letter. Upon receipt of a demand letter, read it thoroughly. This is where Medicare states why they believe they are due money back, and it will include the timeframe you have to respond. If you have general questions about the timeframes,

---

Medicare Overpayments   MLN Fact Sheet

OVERPAYMENT DEFINITION

A Medicare overpayment is a payment that exceeds amounts properly payable under Medicare statutes and regulations. When Medicare identifies an overpayment, the amount becomes a debt you owe the Federal government. Federal law requires the Centers for Medicare & Medicaid Services (CMS) to recover all identified overpayments.

Medicare overpayments commonly occur due to:

* Incorrect coding
* Insufficient documentation
* Medical necessity errors
* Processing and other administrative errors

OVERPAYMENT COLLECTION PROCESS

You must report and return a self-identified overpayment to Medicare as outlined in Section 1128J(d) of the Social Security Act (the Act) within:

* 60 days of overpayment identification
* 6 years from overpayment receipt, generally referred to as the "lookback period"
* If applicable, the cost report due date

When an overpayment is $25 or more, your Medicare Administrative Contractor (MAC) initiates overpayment recovery by sending a demand letter requesting repayment.

Figure 13.3   MLN Fact Sheet: Medicare Overpayments

Medicare provides the chart shown a Figure 13.4 as an overpayment timeline reference guide.

For more information on Medicare's overpayment requirements, navigate to www.cms.gov and refer to MLN Fact Sheet ICN 006379.[6]

DEBT COLLECTION TIMEFRAMES

The following chart shows the overpayment debt collection activities timeframe. It describes how overpayments subject to the Limitation on Recoupment collection differs. It also notes when an action may not apply if an overpayment is in an excluded status (for example, a requested or approved ERS, appeal, or bankruptcy).

Overpayment Debt Collection Activities

Timeframe	Activity
Day 1	MAC sends an overpayment determination demand letter within 7 calendar days.
Days 1–16	**MAC begins immediate recoupment** by Day 16 if you request it.
Day 15	Last day to submit a rebuttal.
Day 16	**MAC begins standard Part A overpayment recoupment** not subject to Limitation on Recoupment or in an excluded category.
Day 30	Last day to pay in full to avoid interest accrual. Last day to request an appeal and stop overpayment recoupment subject to Limitation on Recoupment. If you file an appeal after Day 30 and by Day 120, your MAC stops recoupment **subject to limitation on recoupment** when it receives and validates your appeal but will not refund money already recouped.
Day 31	**Interest accrual begins** for unpaid overpayments by Day 30.
Day 40	Last day to pay overpayments in full before recoupment begins, subject to Limitation on Recoupment, unless it is in an excluded category.
Day 41	**MAC begins standard overpayment recoupment,** subject to Limitation on Recoupment, unless overpayment is in an excluded category.
Days 61–90	MAC sends Intent to Refer (ITR) letter for eligible delinquent debts.
Day 90	MAC attempts to contact you by phone if the debt is 60 days delinquent and not in a status excluded from referral to the U.S. Department of the Treasury (the Treasury).
Day 120	Last day to submit initial appeal request.
Days 126–150	Debt referred to the Treasury according to timelines specified in the Digital Accountability and Transparency Act (DATA).

Figure 13.4   MLN Fact Sheet: Debt Collection Timeframes

Patient Credit Balances

Patient overpayments create credit balances and can occur for any number of reasons. The front desk may have collected a copayment when one wasn't required (i.e., a physical appointment). Or the patient may be unaware they've met their maximum annual out-of-pocket amount and pays a copay. The patient's secondary insurance could pick up a remaining deductible balance the patient assumed wouldn't be covered, or perhaps the patient paid on a denied claim only for the denial to be overturned and the claim to be paid by insurance. Regardless of the reason, the practice needs to return patient credit balances to the patient. Figure 13.5 is a sample patient credit balance report.

Patient	Accounct No.	Charges	Receipts	Balance
Smith, Jones A.	1112345	500.00	750.00	250.00
Thompson, Anna	1112345	125.00	175.00	50.00
Zed, John	1112345	50.00	100.00	50.00
Total Accounts	3	675.00	1025.00	350.00

Figure 13.5   Sample Patient Credit Balance Report

In the above table, we identify three patients with credit balances. Now that these overpayments have been identified, three things must happen:

1. Verify the accuracy of the credit balance.

2. Notify the patient of the credit balance.

3. Refund the patient to resolve the credit balance.

If the patient has an upcoming appointment for which there will be a balance to offset, many practices keep the credit and simply notify the patient. Regardless of the patient's position on the credit balance or scheduled upcoming appointments, credit balances need to be resolved in 30-60 days. If the patient will not be seen in that time frame, then the practice should issue a refund to the patient and document thoroughly.

Process to Minimize Credit Balances

It is in the practice's best interest to reduce the number of accounts that end up with a credit balance. Analyze the trends of your practice's overpayments (i.e., refunds/overpays, posting errors, missing or voided charges). It can help you confirm you have an issue with overpayments and assist in beginning to address any gaps or blind spots in your processes.

If you have identified this as an issue, create a correction plan to prevent further credit balances from being created. This will involve performing an onsite review of the systems currently in place to calculate, confirm, and post payments at the front desk. Also review the process for payment posting and reconciliation of balances due.

Assess your internal protocols for credit balance resolution and establish a threshold for private pay balances. For example, your organization may determine that balances due to the practice under a certain amount (i.e., $5) due to practice from patient can be adjusted off without additional research. Once the policy is approved and established, educate staff on the process for review and processing of credit balances for both federal and commercial insurances as well as self-pay.

Make sure to train and educate staff on how credit balances will be corrected. You can assist in ensuring the correct documentation is gathered by creating a template for all refunds that includes a detailed narrative and back-up documentation explaining how the credit balance occurred. This will service as complete documentation for the practice on each refund and, usually, there is a location this can be housed within the PM system. The basic protocol for each credit balance is to confirm the refund is due and to whom, issue the refund, and thoroughly document.

Depending on the size of the organization, the finance department may need a separately signed document to attach to the refund payment. A sample form has been included as Appendix F.

Claims Management

The claims management process sets the practice up for payment or denial. As has been emphasized before, scrub claims prior to submission to avoid denials. Having a carefully managed process for verifying insurance and all other claims requirements is essential to denial prevention.

When addressing claims denials, consider the following potential causes: insufficient bill edits, claims never getting to clearinghouse, claims never getting from the clearinghouse to the insurance company, claims sent to wrong address/unit, and claims not submitted within timely filing windows. If none of these appear to be the culprit, assess for incorrect diagnosis codes, excluded procedure codes, or incorrect modifier usage.

Claims/Error Strategy

Always review the billed reports and provide necessary documents when requested. Reviewing the reports from the clearinghouse is a critical step toward understanding and mitigating challenges that exist. It is worthwhile to calculate the time lapse from the clearinghouse to the insurance company and discuss any significant delays with your clearinghouse account representative.

Have a process for taking immediate action on denied claims and document the outcomes for future reference. When reimbursement is recouped or retracted, it's important to respond in a timely fashion and to include all pertinent information available for that date of service.

Promissory Estoppel

Promissory estoppel is a legal action that allows a promise to be legally enforceable. We've all heard the statement from insurance companies that, "This is not a guarantee of benefits." However, if the information they have provided to a practice causes a loss (say in payment for services) because the practice relied on that promise, promissory estoppel prevents the "promisor" from neglecting their promise. That promise does not require a formal contract to be enforced by law.

States may have promissory estoppel guidelines, so always check your state's laws. Overall, consider the following elements and legal terminology when deciding whether to use promissory estoppel to appeal denials:

1. **Promisor.** Entity or individual (the insurer) that made a promise to the Promise (the practice) that caused the Promisee to take action on that promise.

2. **Reliance.** Promisee relied on the promise of the Promisor

3. **Detriment.** The Promisee reasonably relied on the promise from the Promisor and, as a result, suffered some loss or worse position.

4. **Unconscionability.** it is extremely unfair that the insurer did not keep its promise.

5. **Relief.** What the Promisee seeks in asking the promisor to fulfill the promise.

SHOUT OUT GUY

In my own career, I've used promissory estoppel to have denials overturned. One instance was when my staff verified insurance and the payer's website showed that the patient was active on the date of service, provided a copay for specialist services, and no termination date of benefits. Luckily for us, we uploaded a print screen of the payer's website data to the patient's record. Eventually, we received a denial for the patient not having active coverage. We relied on the information we received from the payer's website. Since we were participating with the patient's insurance, we only collected the copayment as per the website data. Had our practice been aware that the patient's benefits were inactive, we would not have relied on the insurance verification information and would have collected the full balance at the time of serve. We were harmed in this situation by only being able to receive a copayment (since the patient refused to pay anything else) and the payer denied the claims. After going through the appeals process, I invoked promissory estoppel and received full claim payment.

As with most legal matters, a practice's ability to recover from an insurer that refuses to pay depends upon specific facts, including, perhaps, the terms of the patient's and the practice's contract with the insurer (if it is in network) and the laws of the jurisdiction where the practice is located. No two cases are the same.

In addition to promissory estoppel (sometimes called *equitable estoppel*), there are several other legal theories that may be available and appropriate to pursue payment. There are two different contract-based claims. A practice may be able to claim that, by refusing to pay, the insurer breached its contract with the practice. Or, through an assignment from a patient that transfers to the practice the patient's rights against the insurer, a practice may be able to collect by claiming that the insurer violated its contract with the patient.

A misrepresentation claim could assert that the insurer either negligently or intentionally made a false statement to the practice knowing that the practice would rely on the statement and provide services for the insured. In some states there may be a claim that a retroactive refusal to pay is an illegal unfair and deceptive trade practice.

Two practical takeaways from all of this are: (1) try to negotiate to include in insurance contracts a promise that once authorization has been received, retroactive denial is not allowed; and (2) get insurance authorization in writing (a screenshot can suffice if nothing else is possible or practical) and, when appropriate, a written assignment of benefits from the patient.[7]

Stephen H. Kaufman, Partner, Wright, Constable & Skeen, LLP

The Revenue Cycle Process

It is beneficial to have documented policies and procedures for each phase of the revenue cycle. This allows for accountability and staff's ability to use as a reference document as needed.

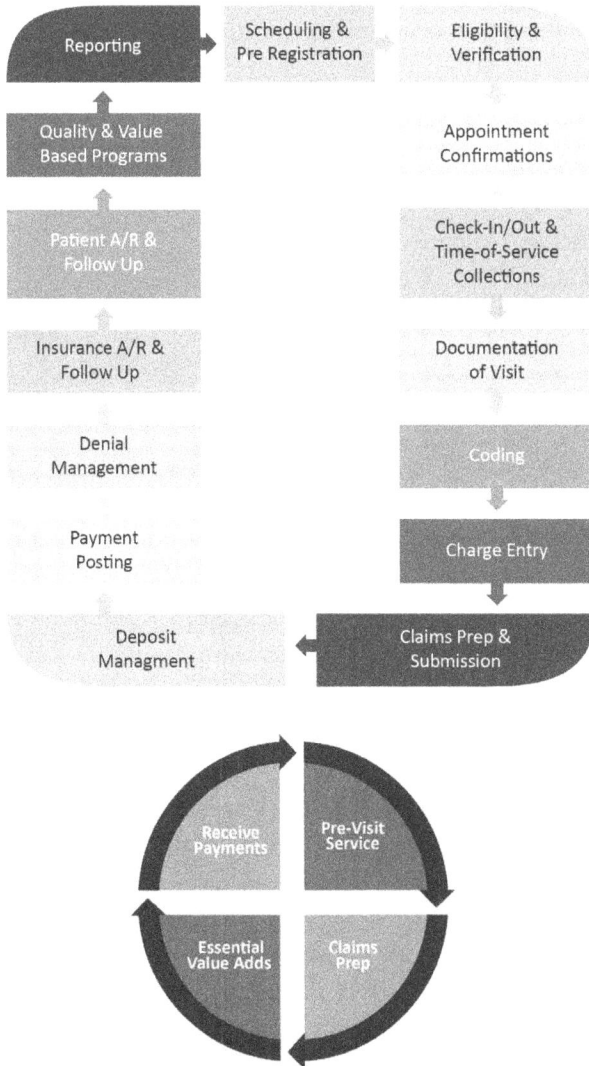

Figure 13.6   The Revenue Cycle Process

Billing Processes

Billing staff work best when they are aware of company expectations regarding the management of the billing process. Open communication between the billing, front desk, and clinical staff is vital to the overall success of RCM. Much of the billing process is impacted by the pre-visit services that include scheduling & Pre-registration, insurance eligibility and benefits verification, appointment confirmations, and check-in.

Billing processes also include evaluation and charge capture, authorizations, claims processing, claims scrubbing, claims transmission, (24-hour) review billed reports, (24-hours) review acceptance report, (7 days) A/R follow-up, payment posting, patient statements and collections.

Leverage detailed processes to assign billing staff to each process and to ensure specific tasks are being carried out accurately and timely.

Medicare Claims Processing

Medicare claims have some of the most complex policy and reimbursement guidelines.[8] Staff assigned to Medicare accounts should be well-versed in these regulations and have solid processes for denial mitigation in place to avoid and manage denials. The Medicare claims process is a bit different than the process listed above. It includes claims submission (within 48-72 hours), claims processed by clearinghouse (within 72 hours), claims forwarded to carrier, carrier download and scrubbing, 1st level rejections, claims processing, 2nd level rejections, more claims processing, 3rd level rejections, claims adjudication, and payment.

LIGHTBULB To optimize revenue, consider holding payers' feet to the fire regarding their payment of late fees on claims that they failed to pay in a timely manner. The late fee payment guidelines and a payment structure are in your participation agreement. If they are not, ask for this information prior to contract execution. Although individually the payments aren't much, over time, these payments add up. Not following up on these payment opportunities sends an industry-wide message to payers that non-payment of late fees is acceptable.

Chapter 13 Knowledge Check

Insurance A/R Follow-Up

Question #1:

A/R stands for _____

Question #2:

True or False? Credit balances can be kept by the practice in the form of a bonus.

Question #3:

For 120 days+ A/R Aging, _____% or higher of total A/R is a sign that there may be issues to resolve.

Question 4:

Credit balances are also referred to as _____.

Question 5:

Promissory estoppel is _____

Answers:

Q1: Accounts Receivable,
Q2: False,
Q3: 20%,
Q4: Overpayments,
Q5: a legal action that allows a promise to be legally enforceable.

Endnotes

1. https://www.experian.com/assets/healthcare/white-papers/white-paper-pre-reg-working-the-healthcare-revenue-cycle.pdf

2. Affordable Care Act, §6402(a) (42 U.S.C. §1320a-7k(d)(1) for more information

3. https://www.cms.gov/Outreach-and-Education/Medicare-Learning-Network-MLN/MLNProducts/Downloads/OverpaymentBrochure508-09.pdf

4. HFMA Credit Balances: https://hfma-nca.org/wp-content/uploads/2018/03/Monday-415-Legislative-Compliance-Credit-Balance-Resolution.pdf

5. Credit Balances OIG: https://oig.hhs.gov/oas/reports/region4/41404029.pdf

6. https://www.cms.gov/Outreach-and-Education/Medicare-Learning-Network-MLN/MLNProducts/Downloads/OverpaymentBrochure508-09.pdf

7. Book quote provided by: *Stephen H. Kaufman, Partner, Wright, Constable & Skeen, LLP*

8. https://www.cms.gov/Regulations-and-Guidance/Guidance/Manuals/Downloads/clm104c23.pdf

Chapter 14

Patient A/R & Follow Up

Following up on patient A/R includes review and management of self-pay claims and patient statements. If the organization works with an external bad debt agency, then optimization is crucial. It is in the practice's best interest to have standard, documented guidelines that dictate company policy on patient balances both in and out of collections, patient copays, payment arrangements, and financial hardship qualifications.

Patient Statements

A practice coordinating and mailing its own patient statements pays approximately $1.00 a statement. That cost includes labor, supplies, and postage. According to the *2013 Instamed Trends in Healthcare Payments Annual Report*, 78% of providers indicated they typically mailed more than one paper statement to collect a patient's payment.

"High Cost of Mailing Patient Statement," *NTC Healthcare*, May 27, 2014.

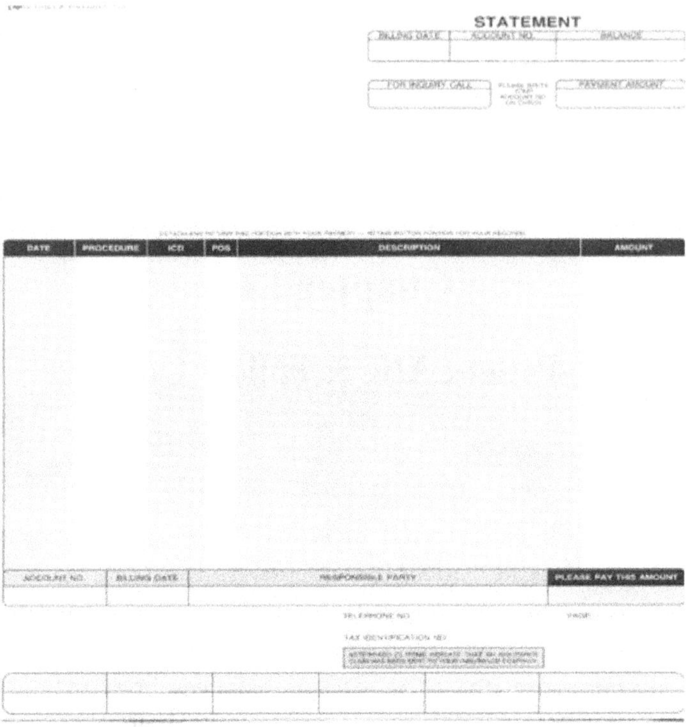
STATEMENT

DATE	PROCEDURE	ICD	POS	DESCRIPTION	AMOUNT

PLEASE PAY THIS AMOUNT

Figure 14.1 Sample Patient Statement Document

Consumer Healthcare Spending Is on The Rise

According to a 2014 article in the *New York Times*, "The report from PriceWaterhouseCooper's Health Research Institute forecasts medical cost growth of 6.8 % overall in 2015."[1]

For calendar year 2015, a *high deductible health plan* is defined under § 223(c)(2)(A) as a health plan with an annual deductible that is not less than $1,300 for self-only coverage or $2,600 for family coverage, and the annual out-of-pocket expenses (deductibles, co-payments, and other amounts, but not premiums) do not exceed $6,450 for self-only coverage or $12,900 for family coverage.[2]

Table 14.1 below outlines some of the differences among the different consumer-driven healthcare payment models. These are types of accounts a patient can open to preserve funds that will be directed to healthcare payment and receive consideration under the U.S. tax code. It is useful for staff to be able to educate patients about these options they may have access to implementing, particularly for expensive healthcare like surgery.

Table 14.1   Consumer Driven Healthcare Payment Models

	Health Savings Account (HSA)	Health Reimbursement Account (HRA)	Flexible Spending Account (FSA)
How is it funded?	Employee or employer funded	Employer funded only	Funded by employee through employer
How is it taxed?	Funded pre-tax Must be reported on employee's taxes	Does not tax employee on funds reimbursed from employer	Funded pre-tax through payroll
Year-End Keep/Lose?	Funds roll over annually	Funds rollover at employer's discretion	Limited funds may rollover at employer's discretion
Owned by	Individual participant	Unused dollars owned by employer	Owned by employer
Can be used for	Qualified medical expenses only	Qualified medical expenses only	Qualified medical expenses and qualified non-medical expenses
Other Details	Set up at a bank Additional tax advantages For use with high-deductible plans		

Workforce Education on Patient Collections Practices

Fair Debt Collections Practices Act

The Fair Debt Collections Practices Act (FDCPA) was passed by Congress and signed into law by President Jimmy Carter in 1977. It was originally enforced by the Federal Trade Commission (FTC). The FTC also established guidelines for acceptable debt collection practices. With the passage of the Dodd-Frank Wall Street Reform and Consumer Protection Act in 2010, the Consumer Financial Protection Bureau (CFPB) was established. It is the CFPB that now establishes guidelines for acceptable debt collection practices, while both the FTC and CFPB have enforcement responsibilities for the FDCPA. This law is what prohibits debt collectors from calling at 2:00 in the morning, among other guidelines.[3]

This law only applies directly to "debt collectors," and any creditor who is attempting to collect debts for itself and under its own name is not considered a "debt collector." Nonetheless, any employees responsible for collecting debt on behalf of the practice should be educated on FDCPA, as these standards provide a good basis for collections decision making. Employees should also be educated in consumer healthcare payment options that provide lines of credit for large expenses, like surgeries.

Each practice should establish documented business processes and workflows that outline how patients accounts are located, notated, updated, and collected on. These workflows and processes should also review the techniques and scripting for collections practices, as well as the organization's policy on non-payment consequences.

In-Person Patient Collections Discussions

Many employees do not feel comfortable collecting past-due balances from patients. The key in these situations is to thoroughly train and educate your staff in "how" and "why." By educating the front desk and any reception staff on the importance of collections and the role they play in the overall revenue cycle, you will empower them to act effectively on behalf of the practice while maintaining good relationships with the patients.

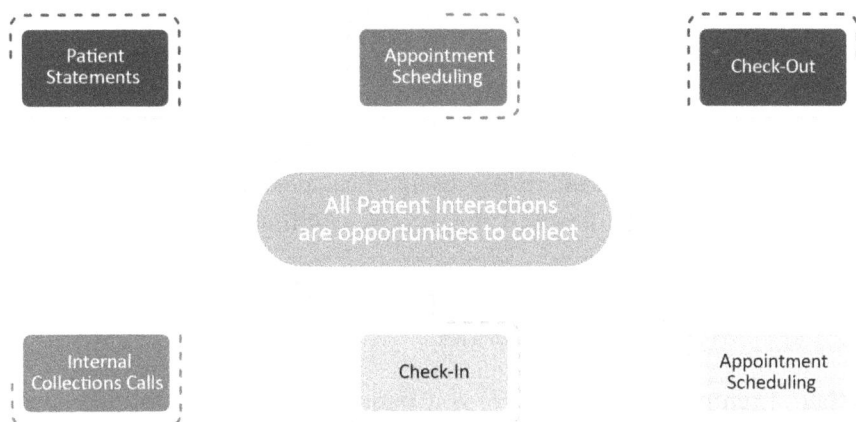

Figure 14.2 Opportunities for Notifying Patients of Balances Owed

For face-to-face collections, make sure staff is aware of how to implement appropriate HIPAA privacy considerations. If the lobby is too small to provide privacy, meet with patients in an empty exam room or quiet office to discuss their balances.

During the conversation remove the provider from the discussion. It is ideal if you can offer multiple payment options, explain balances, and obtain a commitment for payment. It is also very important not to appear confrontational, as many patients will find this topic emotional. Conversations can be improved by stating facts, staying objective, and leaving the patient with something in writing that outlines their financial obligations to the organization.

HIPAA-Compliant Communications

When patients are not available for face-to-face discussions, there must be alternative methods of reaching out. Before leaving messages for patients, the practice must obtain and document the patient's consent to do so and at which phone number that is acceptable. Even with the patient's consent, the practice should take caution to only leave the minimum information necessary. Consider leaving the provider's name as opposed to the practice name, avoid unsecured emails as a form of communication, and ensure that patient communications are a focal point during the annual security risk assessment.

Remove Payment Obstacles

Patients may be reluctant to pay their bills; most who do not work in healthcare do not understand the complex billing environment or the difficulties associated with obtaining payment for services. As such, paying their healthcare responsibilities falls to the wayside or becomes secondary to other patient priorities.

When attempting to collect from a patient, it is very helpful to have as many methods of payment available as possible. At a minimum, the practice should accept cash, money orders, and credit cards. As there is a generation of individuals who still prefer to write checks, consider accepting those as well. It is also convenient if you can offer payment processing through the patient portal. Make sure staff have information on the nearest ATM handy. The practice can also offer automated payment deductions for large balances.

If several methods of payment are available to the patient, you remove excuses from the patient, thereby increasing your chances of collection.

Automated Payment Options

Accepting electronic and automated payments means greater options for patients and faster receipt of revenue for the practice. Consider the use of credit card swipers at the front desk, as well as in the billing department. By linking the credit card swipers/machines to the PM software, some PM systems can auto-post to the patient's account with secured receipt transmission. This is often the case with patient portals as well. Automated posting and receipt generation can save several steps for employees.

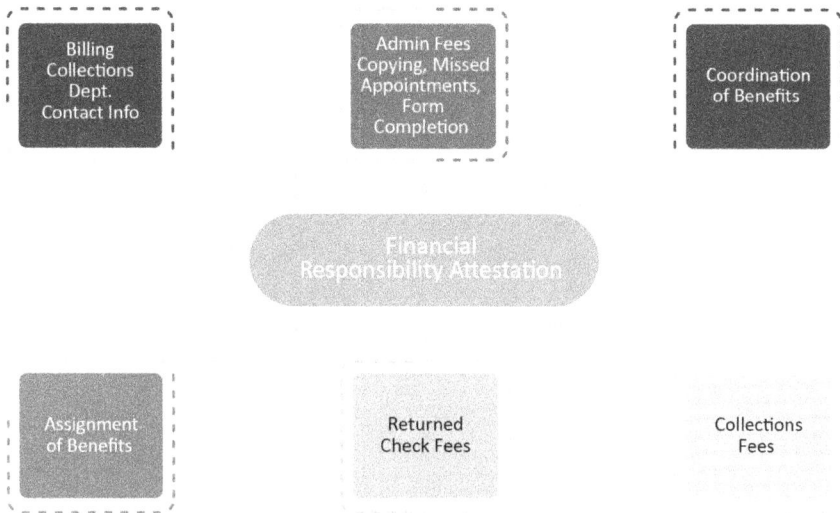

Figure 14.3   Financial Policy Content

Fee Schedule and Allowed Amounts

As discussed earlier, the *fee schedule* is the charge and the *allowed amount* is the contracted payment. You will want to make sure staff are aware of practice pricing and payer allowable amounts. See Table 14.2 for a simple example. This will engage them in spotting payment errors. Provide your front desk staff the tools and training to assist in estimating the cost of care. To support cost estimates, utilize the clearinghouse and obtain real-time claim adjudication for time-of-service collections.

Notifying patients of a prospective financial responsibility ahead of a costly procedure can result in faster reimbursement. This also grants practices an opportunity to collect the allowable amount of unsatisfied deductible prior to the procedure. This is a process often employed at dental offices and Ambulatory surgery centers (ASCs), but it is little used in private practice. It is generally easier to collect from the patient prior to the services being rendered, which is why this process should be considered.

Table 14.2   CPT® Selection Frequency Charge versus Allowable

CPT®	Description	Charge	Payer 1 Allowable	Payer 2 Allowable
99213	Est Level 3	$100.00	$50.00	$75.00
99214	Est Level 4	$150.00	$75.00	$95.00
99215	Est Level 5	$200.00	$95.00	$115.00

Bad Debt

Bad debt is the go-to industry term for patient A/R that is past due. Define standard internal criteria for when accounts should be considered bad debt and what next actions should be taken. Most organizations outsource their bad debt collections to a collections agency.

If outsourcing, make sure to establish criteria that define success for your organization. For example, establish thresholds between payment plan and write-off, set the terms by which bad debt should be escalated to a legal case, and provide parameters of discounts for the agency to negotiate within. The agency will define what demographic or financial data is needed to transfer an account, but the practice should define the consequences of non-payment.

Keep in mind that once an account has been sent to collections, a contingency fee on any payments made thereafter would apply, even if the patient pays the practice directly.

Collection Agencies

Selecting a collection agency can be challenging. It's important to remember that what you're looking for is an agency who will become a partner in your revenue collection process. In addition to researching capabilities, past performance, and tactics, you will want to review the culture of the organization. Do they align with the community that you support? Do they align to your visions of collection? Will they be aggressive enough in collecting your money? Will they be too aggressive? These are just some of the questions you will want to ask your prospective vendors.

It's not all about the relationship. You don't want an agency that is great on the phone with you but horrible at collecting your money. Look at specific KPIs and practices that you can assess across all the vendors you evaluate.

Collections KPIs and Practices

Recovery Rate

The recovery rate reflects what percentage of total debt they recover on average. This is usually the most marketed facet of collections agencies because it's how they score themselves against each other.

Time to Collect

This KPI may be included when they answer about recovery rate but, if not, be sure to ask.

Services Offered

Some common services include soft-collect, hard-collect, and litigation. Think of the first two as, "Hey, did you forget you owe us money?" and "All right, enough is enough, we want our money."

Legislative Knowledge

As mentioned earlier, there are strict regulations regarding the FDCPA (also see Chapter 15). Are they well-versed in these practices? How often are staff educated?

Fees

How do they set their fees? Is it based upon what they recover? Are there different rates for soft-collect? What do they charge for litigation services? Is it a flat fee or a percentage?

Location

Are they a local company? Some practices prefer an agency with a local area code calling their patients. Others may prefer an agency with national collection experience. Identify where they are calling from and ask to listen to sample calls if possible.

Tactics

Identify how the agency intends to contact your patients. Request samples of their mailouts, phone scripts, and email notifications where available. Ask outright if they threaten patients. There are agencies who believe that threatening tactics are the most appropriate. In most cases, this does not equate to a higher recovery rate, and it will breed discontent in the community toward your practice.

Method of Upload

You will need to identify what methods are available to send patients to collections. Does the agency integrate with your practice management system? Do you need to upload a secure file to their website?

Method and Frequency of Reporting

Make it clear that you demand transparency in collections. Turning over the accounts to collections shouldn't reduce your visibility into the collection's performance.

Methods of Payment

Ensure that patients have several options to pay their outstanding balance and confirm the process for patients who wish to pay the practice directly for an account in collections.

Credit Reporting

Do they report patients to credit bureaus upon receipt of debt? If so, do they also regularly report when patients have absolved their debt?

Association Memberships

Do they participate with ACA International? ACA International is a global non-profit group that represents collections agencies of all kinds and require their members to strictly abide by federal law as well as their own code of ethics.

Contract Terms

How long is their standard agreement? Is it negotiable? What are the exit terms and time periods? How long prior to termination must you notify them? What is the method by which they will return the accounts to you?

Global Payment: Some services require a period of monitoring afterward. Any services rendered the period thereafter are bundled into the initial payment. This is referred to as a global payment of services.

Evaluating Your Collection Agency

You should review the performance of your collection agency annually at minimum. When evaluating, do not rely solely upon the metrics they provide. Do your own analysis to confirm. Below are three commonly used formulas to use in your analysis:

Gross Collections Formula = Total Collected ÷ Total Debt Sent for Collections

This is a quick and dirty analysis: what did we send you to get and what of that did you get?

Net Cost of Collection Formula = Total Collected – Fees ÷ Total Debt Sent for Collections

This is a net profit analysis against your debt collections program. Are you paying more to collect your money than you are receiving? Is there a large-enough margin that there aren't concerns going forward?

Net Collections Formula = Total Collected ÷ Total Collectable Sent for Collections

This is a bit more complex. What did we send you to collect? What of that was collectable? What portion of what was collectable did you get? For example, if a patient files for bankruptcy, collections attempts should cease in order to follow the bankruptcy proceedings instead. In these situations, the collections agency is not at fault because that debt is uncollectable.

If you perform your due diligence up front and regularly communicate with and evaluate your collections agency, you can build a long-term relationship. If you do build a long-term relationship, then make sure that you compare your annual findings across the previous 3-5 years. If you notice a trend in decreased performance, then you may need to reevaluate your relationship.

✎ Chapter 14 Knowledge Check

Patient A/R & Follow-Up

Question #1:

Circle One: Educating staff on and abiding by FDCPA **is/is not** optional

Question #2:

Gross Collections Formula =_____

Question #3:

HRAs are funded by _____

Answers:

Q1: Is Not,
Q2: Total Collected ÷ Total Debt Sent for Collections,
Q3: Employers

Endnotes

1. *New York Times, June 24, 2014*

2. *IRS - 26 CFR 601.602: Tax forms and instructions*

3. Kevin M. Lewis. "The Fair Debt Collection Practices Act: Legal Framework," Congressional Research Service In Focus, June 10, 2019, https://fas.org/sgp/crs/misc/IF11247.pdf

Chapter 15

Reporting

For better or for worse, healthcare is inundated with data. Any practice is likely to have multiple sources of information with significant volumes of potential data to assess. Make sure you focus on data that is useful for decision-making that will improve patient care, streamline processes, maintain compliance, and improve the revenue cycle.

Deciding to dive into data analysis is a great opportunity to leverage the full capabilities of your EHR and PM software. There's no additional cost associated to accessing these internal resources, but keep in mind that the data extracted from these resources are only as good as the information that is entered. This is where taking proactive steps to effectively manage your data will really reward the practice.

Data Management

Data that benefits from active management to ensure it is accurate and up to date includes patient registration data, visit documentation, and claims data. Management of the data associated with these processes is critical to success.

> Claims data management is extremely important, as it directly effects healthcare organization's cash flow. Proactively managing denials, time to pay, payer

mix, and contractual allowances enables healthcare organizations to know where they stand today and areas they need to improve for the future. Additionally, a strong claims data management analytics solution provides healthcare organizations with the most impactful pieces of data to leverage when re-negotiating payer contracts.[1]

Craig Christenson, H4 Technology

Let's breakdown common software features that house useful data and utilize technology to streamline operations:

Appointment Scheduling

This report provides data on appointment adherence, quantity of visits, and the number of productive days by provider.

Kept, Canceled, and Missed Appointments

Assessing the data around kept, canceled, and missed appointments allows practices several opportunities to improve processes. The practice can follow up with patients who may have missed an appointment to reschedule. for the practice can begin tracking of habitual appointment no-shows. A report showing canceled appointments can be used to charge cancellation/no-show fees if the practice's notification policy wasn't met.

Number of Visits

This data can be used in several practice ratio calculations that include tracking income generated from patient visits, place of service, and provider productivity.

Provider's Number of Days in Office

Having this information allows for compensation tracking and justification, provider productivity analysis, and determination of provider staffing needs.

Merchant Services

The capability of processing electronic patient payments (i.e. credit card transactions) is not inherent to most EHR/PM systems without a third-party processer known as a *merchant servicer*. The merchant servicer acts as a liaison between the patient's credit card company and the practice by processing the electronic payment; this is known as a *merchant services*.

Electronic receipt of patient payments

Receiving patient payments electronically allows for expedited cash flow for payment of patient balances, development of payment plans, and automated payment posting. Some EHR/PM software include an RCM component. In that case, it is common for the software vendor to charge a percentage of collections. The required amount for a practice to pay will include any payments posted, whether insurance-based or self-pay. Therefore, consider trying to exclude self-pay income from this type of agreement if possible or segment it from other receivables.

Patient Portal

A patient portal facilitates incoming and outgoing patient communications, including healthcare campaigns, patients requests for appointments, prescription refills, and online bill payments.

Patient Registration

Patient registration is probably one of the most important software features as it is the main source of data and is transmitted to other areas of the system to allow for medical record documentation, communication, appointment scheduling, billing, and collections.

Quality Program Dashboards

Proper data management will allow the practice to better select and keep track of progress with Merit-based Incentive Payment System (MIPS) and Alternative Payment Models (APMs) program measures. Many EHR/PM software packages also serve as registries that allow for tracking and reporting of Quality Payment Program (QPP) submission directly in your software. For example, for MIPS 2019, this would include calculations on quality measures (45% of total score), promoting interoperability (25% of total score), improvement activities (15% of total score), and cost data (15% of total score).

A/R Reports

You will want to track aging of balances, claim submission, and payer mix. Since it can take payers 14-45 days to pay, the practice can use these reports to help it avoid aging A/R that is higher than 60 days. Aging A/R that is higher than 60 days is an indicator of a below average collections performance.

Managing KPIs

Utilizing KPIs provides leaders with the tools needed to manage the revenue cycle by utilizing internal data to track, create action plans, and make decisions to improve the financial health of an organization.

Extract KPIs from all available resources including EHR/patient records, coding software, PM software, clearinghouse data, medical societies and organizations, and healthcare facilities

There are many ways to use KPIs for analysis. Enhance the review of providers, productivity, trends and finances by assessing practice KPIs against industry benchmarks. KPIs can be presented in many ways, but the key is to present the right amount of information to the appropriate individuals. Whether that's through graphs, executive summaries, reports, dashboards, or other formats, the key is relevancy and accuracy. Ensure that you have thoroughly vetted and reviewed the KPIs to present and have access to back-up data if needed.

Accuracy is important because KPIs are intended to be used for decision-making. Avoid letting the data get stale, as KPIs can change quickly depending on what is being measured, so the frequency of data extraction and mining should align with that subject matter. Keep in mind that output data is only as valuable as the information put into the system, so data integrity standards are essential. Also of note, KPIs shared once a year may be forgotten, just as KPIs shared daily may be ignored. Frequency should also be matched to the subject matter so that the data received is meaningful and actionable.

Time-of-Service Collections Tracking

This is the amount collected at the time services are rendered / on the date of service. Table 15.1 below is an example TOS collections tracker. Copays listed below are contractual patient obligations. The outstanding balances are amounts owed after insurance has paid their portion or whenever a patient has an out-of-pocket expense. Gather this data to (1) create tracking mechanisms to monitor what was collected vs. what was owed, (2) utilize data to notify patients of out-of-pocket expenses prior to date of service, and (3) track staff time of service collections success and conduct retraining as needed.

Table 15.1   Example Daily TOS Collections Tracker
Calculate the variances daily to identify daily captured or lost revenue opportunities.

Copays Owed	Copays Collected	Variance	Balances Owed	Balances Collected	Variance
$2,500	$2,350	-$150 (Missed Opportunity)	$5,500	$3,500	-$2,000 (Missed Opportunity)

Metrics

Use these metrics for decision-making within your practice. Think of metrics within your own practice and use this tool to apply them to practice.

Unique Patient Visits

The total number of times unique patients had visits with the practice. You can track income and productivity by visit volume. This information is useful to assess:

1. Staffing needs.

2. Exam room utilization.

3. Additional medically necessary services.

4. Productivity and income potential formulas require it.

5. Appointment schedule for optimization.

CPT Code Utilization

Tracking usage and selection of CPT® codes to describe services rendered. Analyze CPT® code utilization by provider, location, timeframe, and payer.

1. Bell curve/coding compliance (use can use AAPC tool to evaluate your utilization as compared to national Medicare averages: https://www.aapc.com/resources/em_utilization.aspx)

2. Medical necessity

3. Clinical Documentation Improvement (CDI)

4. Reimbursement variances by payer

Diagnosis Code Utilization

Understand how often particular diagnosis codes are used to describe illness/injury.

1. Inclusion in wellness and related health campaigns

2. Coding compliance

3. Service complexity

4. Correct sequencing

5. Include 2 or more chronic conditions in CCM program

Patient Zip Code

Geography of patient base in connection to practice location.

1. Marketing

2. Understand payer market for potential expansion of payer participation

3. Consideration of practice expansion

Referring Provider

Indication of the name, specialty and location of providers who are referring to a practice. Number of patients referred by providers.

1. Marketing (without violating Stark or Anti-Kickback Laws)

2. Send appropriate medical records and consultation notes back to referring providers for continuation of care.

Provider productivity

The number of unique patient encounters by each provider in the practice. Compare unique visits to provider's scheduled availability.

1. Provider compensation

2. Manage practice schedules

3. Distribution of practice resources related to supporting providers

Location productivity

The number of unique patient visits by place of service.

1. Site overhead feasibility

2. Site resource distribution

Denial reasons

Communication from payers as to a determination to deny payment of a claim.

1. Identify denial trends to create and implement alternative billing protocols

2. Determine success rate for appeals

3. Create software scrubbing and rules to avoid future denials

4. Determine appropriate use of ABN

Payer mix and income

Volume of beneficiaries seen by practice by individual insurance companies. Percentage of practice revenue by payer. Provides details on payer profitability.

1. Determine continued payer participation.

2. Consider reimbursement increase request.

3. Awareness of administrative burden and cost compared to overall payer income.

4. Awareness of practice income by payer.

5. Compare payer reimbursement to identify lower paying insurance companies to consider renegotiating rates based on practice's value proposition.

6. Develop protocols to address unique payer reimbursement guidelines.

Adjustments

Amount of money written off as not-payable for either contractual or non-contractual reasons.

1. Address write offs that translate into poor collections performance (i.e., timely filing, courtesy, missing referral or no authorization).

2. Compare contractual adjustments with charge amount to determine if charges are equitable.

3. Create rules that require approval for certain adjustment.

Patient Age

The age of active patients in a practice.

1. Perform age based medically necessary services (i.e., Annual wellness visits, preventive services, pediatric care, well-woman services).

2. Track equipment, vaccines and other supply needs.

Gross charges

The amount a practice bills for a specific service offered to patients for a certain timeframe. A Charge Description Master (CDM) houses all the practice's charges by CPT® code.

1. Track fluctuations in charges (high or low) over a certain timeframe.

2. Estimate expected payments-based volume.

Net collections

Payments received after all write-offs.

1. Determine income earned for a specific period.

2. Develop improvements to the overall collections process based on ratios.

Credit balance totals

A patient account has received payment but is not at a zero balance. An error has occurred which skews the account creating a credit.

1. Identify and resolve payment posting errors, overpayments, duplicates, underpayments, COB issue.

2. Initiate refunds.

3. Create and monitor policy to prevent, identify and address and eliminate future credits balances.

Payment posting per payer fee schedule

This provides a method to check payment received against contractually agreed payment amount.

1. Upload payer contract fee schedules (allowable amounts).

2. Identify variances between allowable and received amount.

3. Appeal any errant variances.

4. Develop mitigation policies to prevent errant variances in the future.

5. Create a policy by which this review process regularly occurs.

Take backs

Amount a payer retracts from practice's contracted payments to account for monies owed.

1. Anticipate future payment deductions.

2. Identify overpayment and initiate refund in advance.

Medicare Spending Per Beneficiary (MSPB)

Assesses the average spend for Medicare services for the period immediately prior to, during and following a patient's hospital stay.

1. Review PQRS and QRUR reports.

2. Implement practice improvements (i.e., extended office hours, CAHPS survey, care coordination & transition management.

3. Initiate screenings to include depression, diabetes, and fall.

4. Connect with high risk patients.

Bad Debt

Amounts still outstanding after 120 days of attempts. Sent to agency for recoupment. Contingency fees will apply on each account collected.

1. Review accounts for upcoming appointments prior to sending to bad debt.

2. Compare contingency fee to actual owed balance to determine ROI.

3. Identify and develop action plan to address issues that sent accounts to bad debt

Physician Compensation

Physician expenses are direct physician direct costs which may include salary, health insurance, and retirement.

1. Certain formulas call for the inclusion or exclusion of physician compensation.

Missing Charges

Performed but unbilled services: a missed revenue opportunity.

1. Run reports on testing equipment at the end of the day to capture all tests, labs and related billable services.

2. Have a Certified Coder scan completed progress note to verify the capture and billing of all services.

3. Run missing slips report.

Net Collections

Also referred to as *earned income*, this amount is on the practice's income statement. Ideally, practices would like to collect 100% of owed amounts, but that isn't realistic. Charges are usually set higher than the expected payment amount from insurance companies to account for overhead and other expenses.

Net collections are the amounts received after contractual adjustments (amount practice agreed to accept as a participating provider in a health plan's network), and after refunds and pay back of overpayments. This represents a practice's effectiveness at obtaining collectable amounts.

Inappropriate write offs and credit balances will impact this calculation so be sure to review write off policies as this will skew true net collections rates.

Gross Charges

Amounts billed for a specific period. These charge amounts are based on the practices charge master and do not represent the insurer's allowable amounts.

Adjustments

Combination of required contractual write-offs and potentially incorrect write-offs. This is important data to review, identify any unsanctioned write-offs and appeal.

Formulas

To provide support on using data for decision making, below are formulas to use which calculate varying forms of financial information to manage the financial health of a practice. This data would also be valuable for setting internal benchmarks and goals.

Net Revenue:

$250,000.00 - $100,000.00 = $150,000.00

Gross revenue minus contractual adjustments equals net revenue.

Days in A/R:

The average number of days it takes a practice to collect monies owed.

- Goal: Average performing practices have 40-50 days in A/R.
- Consider calculation to be done in 6- or 12-month increments. This example is for 6 months.

$250,000.00 ÷ 182 = $1,373.63

First calculate average charges in 6 months and divide it by the number of days in 6 months, which will give you your total daily revenue.

$1,373.63 ÷ $70,000.00 = 50.96 or 51 Days

Then take total daily revenue and divide it by amount of aging A/R, which will give you the number of days in A/R.

Average Expense by Patient:

- Goal: _____
- Perform monthly or annually
- Segment by established patient, new patient, or by CPT® code

$70,000.00 ÷ 850 = $82.35

Take the non-physician expense total and divide it by the number of patients to calculate the average expense by patient. In this example, the practice sees 35 patients over 25 days in a month to come up with 850 for a total number of patients.

Net Collections Ratio:

- Goal: _____

$500,000.00 - $14,000.00 = $486,000.00
$850,000.00 - $350,000.00 = $500,000.00

$486,000.00 ÷ $500,000.00 = 0.972 x 100 = 97.2%

To calculate the net collections ratio, take your payments minus the refund/ credit total and divide that number by total charges minus adjustments. Convert that number to a percentage by multiplying by 100.

Net Revenue by Patient:

- Goal: _____
- Calculate monthly or annually
- Segment by established patient, new patient, or by CPT® code

$300,000.00 ÷ 850 = $352.94

To calculate monthly net revenue by patient, take your monthly net collections and divide it by the total number of patients in a month. In this example, the practice sees 35 pts over 25 days in a month.

Days in Receivables Outstanding:

- Goal: 40-45 days

$275,000.00 + $50,000.00 ÷ $7,750 = 41.94 or 42 days

Take the total outstanding and add the A/R total credit balances and divide that by the average daily charge to calculate days in receivables outstanding.

Expense to Earning Ratio:

Costs for running the practice compared to income earned.

- Goal: Lower overhead, higher income.
- Calculate quarterly or annually

$35,000.00 ÷ $100,000.00 = 35%

In this example, quarterly expenses were divided by quarterly net collections to calculate the expense to earning ratio.

In order to run a successful healthcare operation, access to real time data and business intelligent analytics is critical. To me, it all comes down to days cash on hand. This metric is an important measure of hospital liquidity. An organization needs a certain amount to meet the requirement of lenders, rating agencies and others.

The healthcare landscape is very dynamic and is constantly changing. A healthcare system needs to continually monitor its financial performance and assess its strategies relative to what is going on in the marketplace in real time. With the absence of real time data, hospital margins and days cash on hand will continue to decline.[3]

– Tony Tiefenthaler, H4 Technology

Payer Mix

Most income in a typical medical practice will come from insurance payers. Understanding the participation and volume of patients and revenue associated to each payer is a critical KPI for a practice to manage.

Most commercial payer contracts will have unique reimbursement rates. Medicare and Medicaid will have standard rates that are not negotiable. Medicaid MCO's rates are typically based on the respective state's Medicaid fee schedule.

Consider that the same CPT® code could be reimbursed at a different rate and processed under different claims adjudication rules along with individual timelines. These realities force the need to pay attention to payer mix in your practice.

> SHOUT OUT GUY Consider that the same CPT® code could be reimbursed at a different rate and processed under different claims adjudication rules along with individual timelines. These realities force the need to pay attention to payer mix in your practice.

Additionally, many health plans have high deductible plans which impacts patients out-of-pocket expenses for medical services. There are also wellness programs and points patients can earn for participation that could lower their out-of-pocket expenses to providers.

Also, depending on your practice's location; certain payers have unique market share in certain credentialing and payer participation.

Who wants to have a high volume of patients from a specific payer that has low reimbursement with high administrative burden? You won't know if you are in that situation without analyzing your payer mix.

Certain specialties may also have a higher or lower payer mix concentration. Example, cardiologists are likely to have a high Medicare population and pediatricians would not.

Payer Mix

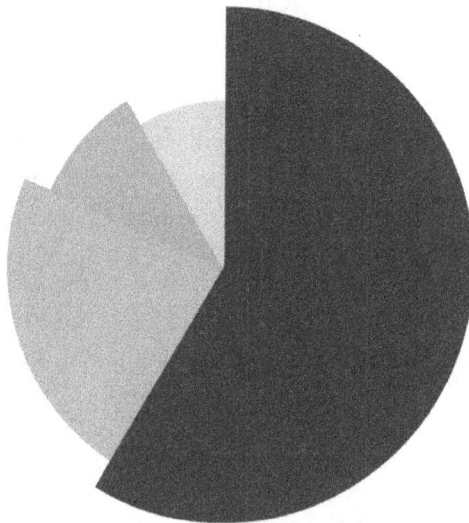

Figure 15.1 Payer Mix

Try to keep up to date contact information for the payers that your practice participates with so you can build report with these individuals. Consider negotiating higher reimbursement rates when possible.

Grouping Payers by Financial Class

When considering how to categorize similar payers to assist with insurance reimbursement and billing management, review similarities of payments, processing structures, volumes and federal programs. Payers that have pay-for-quality metrics (Medicare, Carefirst BCBS, etc.) may be ones you want to compare, and you can use similar dashboards to monitor similar program measures.

Also consider payers with similar payment and claims processing structures. For example, non-participation or TPA plans that allow for balance billing to patients, similar rates, and reimbursement rules. Keep in mind that due to market share or region, there may be a high volume of a specific payer. If that's the case, it is important to track and trend this type of payer individually. It may also benefit to track federal programs like Medicare and Medicaid separately as these have set rates and similar reimbursement guidelines.

Financial Classes

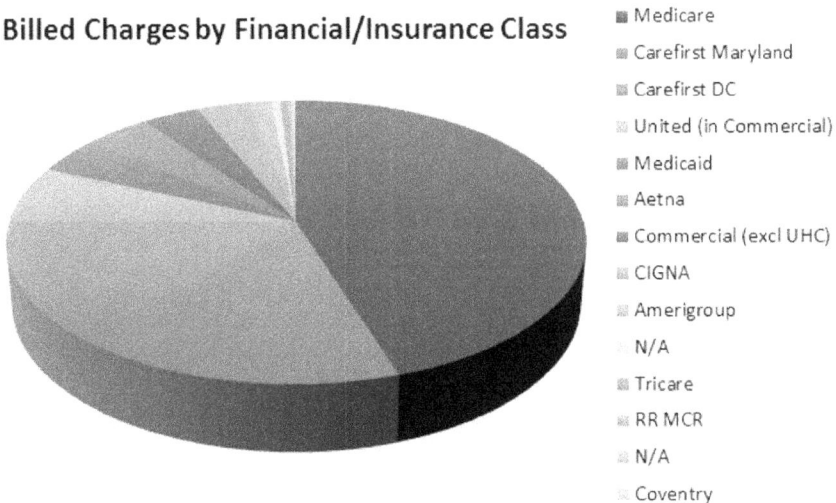

Billed Charges by Financial/Insurance Class

- Medicare
- Carefirst Maryland
- Carefirst DC
- United (in Commercial)
- Medicaid
- Aetna
- Commercial (excl UHC)
- CIGNA
- Amerigroup
- N/A
- Tricare
- RR MCR
- N/A
- Coventry

Figure 15.2   Billed Charges by Financial Class

When assigning a payer to a financial class, stick to one financial class per payer; avoid adding a payer to multiple financial classes. Work with your software vendor to build out financial classes. Tracking billed charges and fee schedules by payer allows a practice to analyze income and forecast revenue. Examples of financial classes include self-pay, Medicare, Medicaid, Medicare Advantage, Medicaid MCOs, Workers' Compensation, managed care, commercial, PPOs, third-party liability and others. It isn't mandatory to set each of these classes up separately, but it does make quite a difference in reporting, so take time to brainstorm where your organization is headed in the future so you can provide an appropriate level of reporting.

Claims Report

Analyzing data in various formats helps to view data in a variety of ways. It also allows one to capture trends without overlooking any. To fully manage claims, net payments and revenues, you'll want to analyze data in a variety of ways.

Review this report and identify discrepancies:

Table 15.2   Claim Report

Claim Count	Net Payment	Insurance Package	% of Total	% Revenue
2,331	$32,300.71	BCBS- PPO	41.08%	8.89%
441	$23,228.25	BCBS- HMO	15.00%	6.39%
411	$21,278.27	SELF PAY	7.24%	5.86%
348	$37,792.20	Aetna	6.13%	10.40%
309	$22,007.63	Medicare	5.45%	6.06%
308	$55,001.14	United Healthcare	5.43%	15.10%
305	$34,496.76	Cigna	5.38%	9.50%
252	$29,159.93	Johns Hopkins - Priority Partners	4.75%	8.03%
237	$32,632.91	Tricare North	4.18%	8.98%

177	$22,002.13	Johns Hopkins - US Family Health Plan	3.12%	6.06%
75	$5,947.37	Workers' comp	2.24%	1.64%
	$315,847.30		100.00%	86.91%

Below are a few key findings from an analysis of the above data:

1. BCBS PPO is 41.08% of the total volume but is only 8.89% of practice revenue.

2. BCBS PPO has the highest claim count but is not the highest source of revenue.

3. United Healthcare is 5.43% of total volume and is 15.10% of total practice revenue.

4. United Healthcare has the 6th highest claim count but is still the top revenue source.

5. Medicare has the 5th highest claim count but has comparable revenue to BCBS HMO.

6. Johns Hopkins – US Family Health Plan the 10th highest claim count but is exactly in line with Medicare's revenues.

7. Johns Hopkins – Priority Partners is a Medicaid MCO, has the 8th lowest claim count but represent revenues higher than that of BCBS HMO, Self-Pay, and Medicare.

8. This practice has a high self-pay population that is uninsured.

9. There are two plan breakdowns for BCBS and for Johns Hopkins.

Table 15.3   Example Fee Schedule

Top 22 CPT® Codes	Fee	Medicare	Payer #1	Frequency	Cost to perform
99203	$ 145.00	$ 117.01	$ 86.09		
99204	$ 220.00	$ 176.87	$ 130.35		
87880	$ 25.00	$ 16.44	$ 10.80		
99214	$ 145.00	$ 115.76	$ 86.93		
99213	$ 100.00	$ 78.84	$ 59.36		
87804	$ 25.00	$ 16.44	$ 10.80		
81002	$ 15.00	Not listed	Not listed		
71020	$ 40.00	$ 30.60	$ 29.28		
87081	$ 25.00	Not listed	Not listed		
73630	$ 45.00	$ 31.91	$ 31.54		
73610	$ 45.00	$ 34.66	$ 37.58		
L2840	$ 65.00	$ 49.85	Not listed		
73140	$ 45.00	$ 34.77	Not listed		
81025	$ 20.00	$ 8.67	$ 6.21		
A6448	$ 10.00	$ 1.29	$ 0.90		
L4360	$ 345.00	$ 276.21	$ 186.00		
73130	$ 45.00	$ 33.88	$ 32.21		
99202	$ 100.00	$ 80.97	$ 59.73		
73562	$ 50.00	$ 39.36	$ 28.52		
12001	$ 125.00	$ 98.27	$ 74.96		
73110	$ 50.00	$ 38.99	$ 28.25		
Q4049	$ 15.00	$ 2.10	$ 2.07		

As you review fee schedule data, be sure to have accurate claims payment information. Request copies of your payer fee schedules and compare them to the amounts posted from EOBs/ERAs in your PM software. If there are variances, then contact your payer to discuss.

A fee schedule gives you the opportunity to review your most frequently used CPT® codes and compare reimbursement for those codes by your top payers. This is also a great opportunity to review your charge amount in comparison to allowable rates by payers as well as analyze the frequency of billed CPT® codes. Use this data negotiate higher reimbursement with payers, determine code selection compliance and capture cost to perform each service.

Revenue Analysis

There are many mechanisms to analyze revenues within a practice. Conducting this analysis in varying ways helps to identify trends or discover opportunities for improvement. For example, determine the number of office visits/services per hour per provider and review the reimbursement per service. Based on the practice's established standard of care, ensure necessary services are being scheduled and performed.

Are all billable services documented and captured? Are the office schedules being maximized to avoid wasted appointment slots?

The simplest forms of analysis include comparing provider productivities and service/procedure productivities. Each of these analyses will give significant insight into the practice's overall perform and each may highlight positive/negative trends for revenue.

Below is a metric that tracks hourly profit by provider. Utilize your practice's data for this calculation.

Table 15.4   Hourly Profit by Provider

Hourly Office Visit Per Provider	Financial Data	
4 L-3 F/U Visits	$373.52	Based on Medicare F/U L3 Visit
PFT x 2 per Hr	$417.95	Based on Medicare PFT Payment
2 Spiros per Hr	$97.72	Based on Medicare Spiro Payment

Hourly Income	$889.19			
Hourly Overhead	$454.27			
Hourly Profit	$434.92			
	x 2080 hrs			
Annual Potential	$904,633.60			

Table 15.5 Additional KPIs:

KPI	Average / Industry Standard	Improvement Needed
A/R over 120 days	12% or lower	20% or higher
Days in Receivables Outstanding	40 – 45 Days	65 or higher
Net Collections	90%	

CPT® Utilization

Reports calculating CPT® utilization assesses the frequency of use by CPT® code and can show trends and unusual activity. This data can be viewed from the perspective of the practice as a whole, or at the individual provider level.

Chapter 15 Knowledge Check

Reporting

Question #1:

KPI stands for _____

Question #2:

TOS stands for _____

Question #3:

Group payers by _____ for reporting analysis

Question 4:

_____ is also referred to as Net Collections.

Question 5:

True or False? Considering it can take payers 14-45 days to pay, you should avoid aging A/R that is higher than 60 days.

Answers:

Q1: Key Performance Indicator or KPI
Q2: Time of Service,
Q3: Financial Class,
Q4: Earned Income,
Q5: True

Endnotes

1. Book quote provided by: Craig Christenson, H4 Technology

2. https://www.aafp.org/practice-management/administration/finances/collection-rate.html

3. Book quote provided by: *Tony Tiefenthaler, H4 Technology*

Chapter 16

Compliance & Risk Management

Developing a company-wide compliance plan is an essential element of the overall risk management of the organization. This includes risk management within the revenue cycle. The penalties and fines associated with noncompliance can be significant enough to threaten the financial solvency of a practice.

Essential elements of revenue cycle management compliance include alignment with these organizations, statutes, and laws, among others:

- U.S. Department of Health & Human Services Department (HHS)
- The Office of the Inspector General (OIG) of the HHS and its *Components of a Compliance Plan*
- HIPAA Compliance
- Red Flag Rule and Compliance
- Fair Debt Collection Practices Act
- Stark Regulations (42 U.S.C.'1395nn)
- Anti-Kickback Statutes
- False Claims Act (31 U.S.C.'3729)
- Federal Criminal False Claims Statutes (18 U.S.C.' 287,1001)

- Civil Monetary Penalties Act (42 U.S.C.'1320a-7a)
- Federal anti-kickback statute (42 U.S.C.'1320a-7b)
- Title XVIII of the Social Security Act
- Patient Protection and Affordable Care Act (Pub. L. No. 111-148, 124 Stat. 119)
- HIPAA (45 CFR Part 164); Fraud and Abuse, Privacy and Security Provisions of HIPAA, as modified by HITECH Act
- Occupational Safety Health (OSH) Act (29 CFR 1910)
- Fraud Enforcement and Recovery Act of 2009
- Clinical Laboratory Improvement Amendments (CLIA) of 1988

Staying abreast of these regulations can seem daunting at first. To make the process easier consider joining an association, like MGMA, that sends news alerts, stays involved in regulatory affairs, and offers participation in education and training. It is also a good idea to engage legal counsel to review your compliance plans and assess whether there are gaps in your processes and policies. If you don't think you need a legal review but you do need advice, consider hiring a subject matter expert to consult on the practice's current or anticipated operations and to identify compliance concerns.

> A good compliance program can help protect practices against charges of improper payments, fraud and abuse, and other potential liability areas. It is important for physicians and staff to understand that an effective healthcare compliance program is a necessary adjunct to quality patient care and promotes better staff communication. Bottomline, it's a win-win for everyone.[1]
>
> [2]*Elizabeth Svoysky, J.D., Vice-President, Risk Management, Medical Mutual Liability Insurance Society of Maryland*

History of Compliance

Compliance mandates in the United States have increased significantly since the early 1990s. Escalating government expenditures led to questions of whether participating organizations were compliant with program requirements.

Whistleblower cases increased. This created a need for additional fraud, waste, and abuse regulations to reeducate participating organizations about compliance.

Each year, the OIG releases a work plan that identifies its areas of focus as a government entity. This is also a way to publicize their efforts.[3] Practices that follow the research, guidance, and outcomes posted on the OIG website can begin to understand the intent behind the office's regulations, as well as its activities.

In addition to the OIG work plan and investigations, HHS created the Health Care Fraud and Abuse Control Program (HCFAC). Both the HHS and the U.S. Attorney General (AG) oversee this organization and have recovered billions of dollars in fraud, waste, and abuse within the healthcare industry.

For the purposes of this book, the focus will stay on compliance concerns as they relate to RCM. Let's start with the primary oversight committee for the healthcare industry, HHS.

Department of Health and Human Services

The mission of the department of HHS is "to enhance the health and well-being of all Americans, by providing for effective health and human services and by fostering sound, sustained advances in the sciences underlying medicine, public health, and social services."[4]

HHS has two divisions, with several departments falling under the umbrella of each one. To view the full list of entities, navigate to www.HHS.gov and search *organization chart*. A sample of the HHS hierarchy is provided.

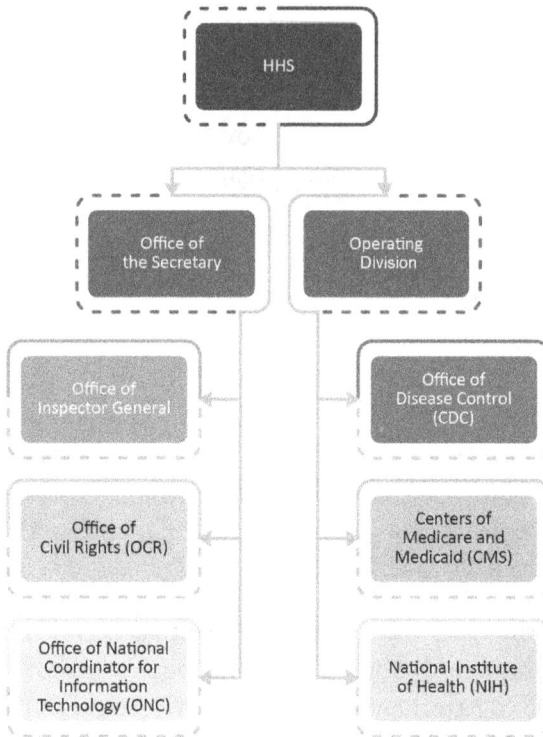

Figure 16.1 Small sampling of HHS departments

Most of the entities under the Office of the Secretary begin with the word *office* to help identify which branch of the HHS they belong to. The purpose behind the Office of the Secretary is to support internal auditing. For example, the OIG ensures compliance with programs created by CMS and the Office of the National Coordinator for Information Technology (ONC) ensures compliance with CMS programs related to information technology.

HHS OIG

As identified above, the OIG operates as part of the HHS and functions to "protect the integrity of Department of Health & Human Services (HHS) programs as well as the health and welfare of program beneficiaries."[5]

To achieve success with this mission, the OIG offers guidance on compliant processes and audits organizations to ensure their alignment with regulations. They also provide a wealth of resources to help practices structure their own compliance policies and to ensure all of their processes are compliant. For example, guidance on creating and maintaining compliance programs is on the OIG website for all facility types and sizes.

It is important that we hire and do business with individuals and organizations that have not been excluded from participating in Medicare, Medicaid, and other federal healthcare programs. The OIG has a List of Excluded Individuals/Entities (LEIE) that informs the public of excluded individuals. The LEIE is updated monthly. An individual or organization appears on this list when the entity has been found to be noncompliant and chooses not to remedy the areas of noncompliance.

Use these step-by-step instructions to search for excluded entities:

1. Navigate to www.oig.hhs.gov.

2. Select the *Exclusions* tab in the top navigation bar.

3. Select *Online Searchable Database* in the left navigation bar.

4. Then enter the name, entity, or entities into the search fields and select Search.

OIG Components of a Compliance Plan

OIG compliance plan components are located on the OIG website.[6] Practices should review their compliance plans annually to ensure they conform to OIG recommendations. Individual and small group physician practices can find compliance plan information by visiting https://oig.hhs.gov/authorities/docs/physician.pdf. Below are a few highlights from an important OIG document about compliance programs and plans. Refer to the original document for further information. The below voluntary standards would apply to every department in the practice or organization, including billing practices.

59434 Federal Register / Vol. 65, No. 194 / Thursday, October 5, 2000 / Notices

Excerpt from "Components of an Effective Compliance Program"[7]

This compliance program guidance for individual and small group physician practices contains seven components that provide a solid basis upon which a physician practice can create a voluntary compliance program:

- Conducting internal monitoring and auditing;
- Implementing compliance and practice standards;
- Designating a compliance officer or contact;
- Conducting appropriate training and education;
- Responding appropriately to detected offenses and developing corrective action;
- Developing open lines of communication; and
- Enforcing disciplinary standards through well-publicized guidelines.

59435 Federal Register / Vol. 65, No. 194 / Thursday, October 5, 2000 / Notices

Excerpt from "B. Benefits of a Voluntary Compliance Program"[8]

The OIG acknowledges that patient care is, and should be, the first priority of a physician practice. However, a practice's focus on patient care can be enhanced by the adoption of a voluntary compliance program. For example, the increased accuracy of documentation that may result from a compliance program will actually assist in enhancing patient care. The OIG believes that physician practices can realize numerous other benefits by implementing a compliance program. A well-designed compliance program can:

- Speed and optimize proper payment of claims
- Minimize billing mistakes

- Reduce the chances that an audit will be conducted
- Avoid conflicts with the self-referral and anti-kickback statutes

59438 Federal Register / Vol. 65, No. 194 / Thursday, October 5, 2000 / Notices

Specific Risk Areas

Excerpt from "1. Specific Risk Areas" [9]

To assist physician practices in performing this initial assessment, the OIG has developed a list of four potential risk areas affecting physician practices. These risk areas include:

1. Coding and billing

2. Reasonable and necessary services

3. Documentation

4. Improper inducements, kickbacks, and self-referrals

Mandatory or Voluntary?

Compliance programs are mandatory for Medicare Advantage (MA) organizations (Part C) and Medicare Prescription Drug Plan (Part D) providers. These guidelines are in the Patient Protection and Affordable Care Act (ACA). Additionally, CMS requires these providers to have a compliance program as a condition of enrollment. The compliance program described within the Federal Register by the OIG, however, is voluntary, but having a program in place is mandatory.

Penalties

Fraud, waste, and abuse is highly penalized. Below are two case examples highlighted in the OIG publication *Avoiding Medicare and Medicaid Fraud and Abuse: A Roadmap for New Physicians.*[10]

Case #1

The Facts: A physician falsely indicated on his provider number application to the CMS that he was running his own practice when, in fact, a neurophysiologist was operating the practice and paying the physician a salary for the use of his number.

The Penalty: $50,000 in restitution

Case #2

The Facts: A physician charged patients, including Medicare beneficiaries, an annual fee. In exchange for the fee, the physician offered: (1) an annual physical, (2) same- or next-day appointments, (3) dedicated support personnel, (4) around-the-clock physician availability, (5) prescription facilitation, (6) expedited and coordinated referrals, and (7) other amenities at the physician's discretion. The physician's activities allegedly violated the assignment agreement because some of the services outlined in the annual fee were already covered by Medicare.

The Penalty: $107,000

Both of the above situations could have been avoided if the practice had enacted and followed a compliance plan using OIG guidelines.

The Health Insurance Portability and Accountability Act of 1996

- Practice goal: reeducate annually or bi-annually with documented employee assessments.

HIPAA includes policies policies and penalties that govern most aspects in health care. The purpose of HIPAA is to protect patient data and to have appropriate technological safeguards in place. The regulations break down into privacy and security policies.

Primary HIPAA components:

- Risk management plan that includes:
  - administrative safeguards
  - technical safeguards
  - physical safeguards
  - general policies and procedures
- Risk assessment that includes:
  - compliance requirement
  - determining vulnerabilities and threats
  - gap analysis
  - remediation based upon actionable items
- Security awareness
  - Must cover four implementation specifications:
    - ✓ security reminders
    - ✓ protection for malicious software
    - ✓ log-in monitoring
    - ✓ password management
  - Should include:
    - ✓ HIPAA privacy and security rules
  - Security risk assessment is an annual requirement.

The full breadth of HIPAA and its implications on practice operations could encompass its own book. For the purposes of this book, we ask you to consider HIPAA as it relates to the revenue cycle management process at your facility:

> In healthcare the cost of a cyber incident is often mistakenly thought to solely mean HIPAA fines. While these can be staggering, the harsh reality for small businesses is that

the costs of a cyber incident may be insurmountable long before regulatory fines and penalties are assessed.

When a cyber incident occurs, IT forensic investigators will need to determine the scope of the breach, while a legal team determines compliance with state and federal laws. Forensic investigators alone charge between $200-$500 per hour to assess your systems and see what kind and how much information has been lost or stolen. Once that information is identified, you may be legally obligated to notify and offer credit monitoring to every individual affected by the breach. Required disclosure to state and federal agencies prolong the investigatory period and disruption.

There is a corresponding negative impact on your bottom line when operation critical systems are down. Restoring and recovering electronic data, computer programs or software after an IT system failure or disruption is not as easy as flipping a switch. Computer programs, including software or applications as a service are generally restored in phases, which can extend the business interruption impact for weeks or months.

Following an incident, additional operational expenses not only include mitigating and remediating the cyber incident, but also business continuity costs, e.g., additional staff may be required to manually perform job tasks normally completed electronically, such as calling prescriptions in to the pharmacy.

No business is immune to the impact of a cyber-attack. Reviewing your cyber risk and any contractual coverage obligations, as well as understanding cyber liability insurance is an essential component of any risk management program.[11]

Jenny L. Jacobsen, JD, Advisor, Risk Management & Regulatory Affairs, SilverStone Group

Penalties

Penalties for noncompliance with HIPAA are based upon the level of noncompliance exhibited:

- Civil monetary penalties range from $100 to $50,000 per violation of each patient record.
- A maximum penalty of $1.5 million per year for identical provisions may be charged.
- Criminal penalties can range to up to 10 years in jail.

Red Flag Rule

- Practice goal: Re-educate annually.

According to the Federal Trade Commission (FTC), "an estimated nine million Americans have their identities stolen each year."[12] The Red Flag Rule exists to help prevent identity theft. It was named this because the general premise is to be on the lookout for "red flags" that the individual is not who he or she says he or she is. To voluntarily protect patients from identity theft, develop a documented program that helps identify potential red flags and dictates next steps to employees. For example, if a patient presents identification that appears to be invalid or is unable to present identification at all, practice employees should recognize this as a red flag and a procedure should be in place for how they should respond.

Make sure to support the program by providing resources to staff that educate them on how to identify red flags. Finally, ensure the program includes policies that will keep it up to date; i.e., an annual review of the Red Flag Program.

Choosing not to implement identity theft protection for your patients may result in nonpayment of claims, patient distrust, and further program audits by federal entities.

Fair Debt Collection Practices Act

- Practice goal: Re-educate annually

Like the Red Flag Program, fair debt collection falls under the supervision of the FTC. To verify that collections activities are fair and reasonable, the Fair Debt Collection Practices Act (FDCPA) was enacted by the 95th U.S. Congress.

The goal of the FDCPA is to prevent abusive collection practices, to ensure that those who are compliant with FDCPA are not competitively disadvantaged, and to encourage consistency in collection practices across the nation.[13] While the Act only applies to debt collection agencies, and not to entities pursuing debt owed directly to them, they nonetheless provide a best-practices model.

Review the comprehensive guidance from the FTC on FDCPA in full.[14] A few of the basic rules it has for debt collection agencies are listed below:

- The Act restricts contacting debtors between 8:00 a.m. and 9:00 p.m. to collect a debt unless they have given you permission to call them at other times.
- The Act stipulates that debt collectors cannot:
  - Threaten violence;
  - Threaten to take property (unless contractually bound and accepted through state law);
  - Use profanity;
  - Call excessively; or
  - Make false statements, for example:
    - ✓ Lie about amounts due, or
    - ✓ Lie about being an attorney.

For more information on FDCPA, visit www.ftc.gov and enter the search term *fair debt.*

The Ethics in Patient Referrals Act of 1989

- Practice goal: Re-educate annually

The Ethics in Patient Referrals Act of 1989, most commonly referred to as the Stark Law, includes the following goals:

1. To prohibit physicians from making referrals for certain designated health services (DHS) payable by Medicare to an entity with which the provider, or the provider's family, has a financial relationship unless an exception applies.

2. To prohibit the entity from presenting claims to Medicare or anyone else for those referred services.

3. To establish specific exceptions and grant the Secretary (of Health and Human Services) the authority to create regulatory exceptions for financial relationships that do not pose a risk of program or patient abuse.

Applicable DHS services include:

- Clinical laboratory services;
- Therapy: physical, occupational, and outpatient speech-language pathology services;
- Imaging services, like radiology radiation therapy services and supplies;
- Durable medical equipment;
- Parenteral and enteral nutrients, equipment, and supplies;
- Prosthetics, orthotics, and prosthetic devices and supplies;
- Home health services;
- Outpatient prescription drugs; and
- Inpatient and outpatient hospital services including those performed at ambulatory surgery centers (ASCs).

Penalties for violating Stark Law range from $15,000 per instance to $100,000 per scheme.

If a provider has a financial interest (ownership, investment, compensation arrangements, etc.) in one of the following, then Stark Law regarding physician referrals should apply:

- Imaging center
- Laboratory
- Ambulatory surgery center
- Hospital
- DME supplier
- Therapy center
- Pharmacy
- Any other business or entity that may lead to referrals of DHS

More information on the Stark Law is available at CMS and at the OIG.

Anti-Kickback Statute (AKS)

- Re-educate annually

Providers are often targets for kickbacks and many times do not fully know the regulations. This can lead them to signing agreements that violate the Anti-Kickback Statute (AKS).

Put simply, in health care *it is illegal to accept referral bonuses, incentives, or inducements of any kind.*

Some examples are straightforward, while others are a little more obscure. Below are some examples of *prohibited* practices:

- Dr. Smith (cardiologist) sends a $50 gift card to Dr. Jones (PCP) for every new patient he refers.
- Dr. Smith rents space in a shared clinic from Dr. Jones. If Dr. Smith refers all his patients to Dr. Jones, Dr. Smith can receive discounted rent up to 10% off.

- Pharmaceutical rep Bob tells Dr. Jones that for every prescription Dr. Jones writes for Bob's company's medications, Dr. Jones will get 10 points. When Dr. Jones gets to 1,000 points, he and his family get a free vacation to Hawaii.

Any purchase plan, discount arrangement, or instance in which cost reimbursement is above fair market value may be an AKS violation.

To avoid AKS violations in your practice:

1. Educate providers and staff in AKS with examples of violations.

2. Encourage providers to bring all potential agreements to management for review for *their* safety.

3. Require pharmaceutical representatives to go through management.

4. Decline lunches and gifts from pharmaceutical reps.

Per the OIG, "Taking money or gifts from a drug or device company or a durable medical equipment (DME) supplier is not justified by the argument that you would have prescribed that drug or ordered that wheelchair even without a kickback." The regulations are very strict, and their goal is to protect patients from services and devices that would not be in their best interest. For more information on AKS, visit www.oig.hhs.gov. There are some excluded *safe harbor* activities that should be reviewed if applicable.

Antitrust Laws

According to the Department of Justice, antitrust laws are put into place to help "contain costs, improve quality, expand choice, and encourage innovation. The Antitrust Division enforces the antitrust laws in healthcare to protect competition and to prevent anticompetitive conduct." An example of an antitrust law violation is healthcare providers sharing charge amounts and insurance reimbursement rates with one another. Speak with your practice's attorney regarding compliance with these laws.[15]

Risk Management

The first step to mitigating risk is to identify that the risk exists. The key to identifying risks is to perform an internal revenue cycle assessment. This means diving into all aspects of the revenue cycle and their methods of management at your facility. Performance of an RCM assessment often identifies issues such as failure to obtain appropriate informed consent, failure to obtain advanced beneficiary notification (ABN), inaccurate billing, rude or inappropriate collections practices, and/or payer enrollment issues.

✏ Chapter 16 Knowledge Check

Compliance and Risk Management

Question #1:

True or False? The Red Flag Program helps prevent identity theft.

Question #2:

True or False? CMS requires providers to have a compliance program as a condition of participation.

Question #3:

True or False? Abiding by the Anti-Kickback Statutes is optional for private practices.

Answers:
Q1: True,
Q2: True,
Q3: False

Endnotes

1. Book quote provided by: Elizabeth Svoysky, J.D., Vice-President, Risk Management, Medical Mutual Liability Insurance Society of Maryland

2. https://oig.hhs.gov/reports-and-publications/workplan/index.asp

3. https://www.hhs.gov/about/strategic-plan/introduction/index.html

4. https://oig.hhs.gov/about-oig/about-us/index.asp

5. https://oig.hhs.gov/compliance/

6. 59434 Federal Register / Vol. 65, No. 194 / Thursday, October 5, 2000 / Notices

7. 59435 Federal Register / Vol. 65, No. 194 / Thursday, October 5, 2000 / Notices

8. 59438Federal Register / Vol. 65, No. 194 / Thursday, October 5, 2000 / Notices Specific Risk Areas

9. https://oig.hhs.gov/compliance/physician-education/roadmap_web_version.pdf

10. Book quote provided by: *Jenny L. Jacobsen, JD, Advisor, Risk Management & Regulatory Affairs, SilverStone Group*

11. https://www.ftc.gov/tips-advice/business-center/guidance/fighting-identity-theft-red-flags-rule-how-guide-business

12. https://www.debt.org/credit/collection-agencies/debt-collectors/

13. https://www.consumer.ftc.gov/articles/debt-collection-faqs

14. https://www.justice.gov/atr/health-care

Chapter 17

Conducting an Internal Revenue Cycle Assessment

An internal revenue cycle assessment should be performed regularly. Some activities, like financial assessments, may require monthly review, while others, like SWOT analyses, are performed annually.

Financial Statements

Accurate financial statements are a primary source of intelligence and information for practice managers. The financial statements provide the information required to assess the current financial health of the organization and to predict its future financial health.

There are a series of reports that should be reviewed regularly. This includes profit and loss statements, the balance sheet, provider productivity, deposits (cash/credit/EFT), cash on hand, aging accounts receivables, and the general ledger for the organization.

Below is a chart that shows suggestions for how often these reports should be reviewed. These may need to be adjusted based upon the size of your organization and the roles/responsibilities of each employee.

Table 17.1   Chart of Suggested Review Cycles

Report	Review Cycle	Comments
Profit & Loss Statements	Monthly	You can review more frequently if preferred, but trends of less than a month at a time may not be fruitful.
Balance Sheet	Monthly	You can review less frequently if your organization rarely effects capital expenditures, loans, or significant changes to assets.
Provider Productivity	Monthly	Depending on the compensation metrics at your organization, this may need to be reviewed more frequently.
Deposits	Daily/Weekly	Deposits should be reconciled every day with totals tracked weekly for trending.
Cash on Hand	Monthly	COH refers to liquid cash as well as assets that can be liquified quickly. If your organization is operating with a thin margin you may want to review this on a weekly or even daily basis.
Aging A/R	Weekly	The billing manager will review this daily. The practice manager should track it weekly to ensure progress is being made and to review any outstanding balances of concern.
General Ledger	Daily	This should be kept current daily and reconciled to match bank transactions if daily access to online banking is available.

Process Assessments

Assessing practice processes should take place annually during the security risk assessment (SRA).[1] When reviewing, you want to make sure that a high-level business process exists for each department and that workflows for each block of the business process also exist.

The U.S. Department of Health and Human Services (HHS) requires all Covered Entities (healthcare providers) that access electronic protected health information (ePHI) to conduct a risk assessment as the first step towards knowing if required safeguards, as specified in The HIPAA (Health Insurance Portability and Accountability Act) Security Rule, are in place. Regardless of the size of the organization or the number of patients, patient records, or how much or how little ePHI is held, a risk assessment needs to be conducted. A checklist will not suffice. An assessment must include a gap analysis, which is overview examination to assess whether certain controls or safeguards required by the Security Rule are implemented, especially from the policy and procedure prospective. A good risk assessment should include a mitigation plan that addresses how to fix or correct moderate to high levels of risk that were discovered. The HIPAA Security Rule states that a risk assessment must be documented and that the overall process of compliance is ongoing, meaning it's not a 'one and be done' deal. The risk assessment will be one of the first documents requested by HHS as part of any breach investigation.[2]

Jay Hodes, President of Colington Consulting

While reviewing the business processes and workflows, look for areas of duplication, gaps in the process/workflow, adherence to process/workflows, and perform a SWOT (strengths, weaknesses, opportunities, threats) analysis.

SWOT Analysis

Some analyses can be annoying to perform but critical to the health of the business to complete. SWOT analyses are much like that. A SWOT analysis helps you identify the strengths, weaknesses, opportunities, and threats within your organization.

The layout of a SWOT organizer does not have to be overly complicated to be effective. There are many resources available online to assist with implementing this process. The most basic format looks something like this:

Strengths	Weaknesses
Opportunities	Threats

Figure 17.1   SWOT Analysis Grid

As with any assessment, it is important to make sure that individuals doing the assessing have actual hands-on participation in these processes. Managers should be involved as well as staff. If a SWOT analysis is performed by individuals too many layers above the individuals who use the workflows in question, then you may fail to gather critical information.

Site Profitability

Site profitability is important to analyze so that you allocate resources properly across your organization and identify any issues impeding profitability as early as possible. You should be able to set your locations up as separate cost centers within your practice management system and accounting software. Work with your accountant to set these up for accurate and meaningful reporting with the opportunity to expand upon existing cost centers as needed.

Below is a snapshot of a sample site profitability tool. This type of evaluation assesses practice site profitability by comparing total patients, charges, adjustments, net collections, and expenses across all locations for three years. Customize this sheet to fit the needs of your organization and review this information annually at minimum.

Table 17.2   Sample Site Profitability Tool

Annual Comparisons	Total Patient Visits		Charges		Adjustments		Net Collections		Expenses	
	Site 1	Site 2	Site 1	Site 2	Site 1	Site 2	Site 1	Site 2	Site 1	Site 2
Prior Year										
Trailing Year										
Year to Date										

Provider Compensation vs. Provider Collections

Structuring provider compensation can involve very challenging and complex metrics. Regardless of complexity, it is critical that you evaluate the net profit of each provider by evaluating the provider's total compensation against the provider's total receipts.

Below is an example of how to set up a basic analysis that compares provider compensation to revenues. Even if you do not employ the use of relative value units (RVUs) as the basis of compensation, they are an excellent weighting tool to review productivity and compensation. At minimum, consider including RVUs as an incentive metric for bonuses or increases.

Table 17.3 Basic Analysis Comparing Provider Compensation to Revenues

Providers	Prior Year			Trailing Year			Year to Date		
	Compensation	RVU	Net Collections	Compensation	RVU	Net Collections	Compensation	RVU	Net Collections

RVU based physician compensation continues to be the most common method when structuring a clinical physician compensation. Why? The physician clinical effort can be directly tied to work RVUs (wRVUs) that are tied to CPT® codes, making the monitoring of productivity fairly simple.

MGMA is one of the best sources available that provides great wRVU benchmark data and is very useful in setting productivity targets.

Although you will need to navigate the nuances of using wRVUs in compensation, it will also provide a solid foundation for basing physician compensation.[3]

— *Kathy Maddock, Maddock & Co.*

Other Assessment Metrics

The other assessment metrics used by your organization will vary based upon the size, setup, and needs of your organization. Other useful assessments for RCM include an analysis of daily charges, credit balances and time line, payer mix, incentive program performance, patient statements, denial rates, and bad debt agency performance. For more information, refer to Chapter 13 for a discussion of credit balances, Chapter 14 for a discussion of patient statements and bad debt, Chapter 12 for a discussion of denials, and Chapter 20 for a discussion of incentive programs.

Daily Charges

Some practices prefer to review the daily charges information each day while others may review it weekly or monthly. A review of daily charges identifies the billable productivity of the entire organization. Like provider productivity metrics, this assessment should review the procedure codes charged out alongside the units, or quantity, of those services billed. The primary difference between a daily charge analysis and a provider productivity analysis is that the daily charge analysis will also capture ancillary services or non-provider charges. For example, in-house pharmacy or laboratory charges should appear in the daily charges review.

Payer Mix

A payer mix is the ranking of insurance providers by charges. For example:

Table 17.4   Example Payer Mix

Cutten Mend Health	$1,500,000	50%
Big Federal Insurance	$1,000,000	33%
Green Tea Health Plan	$ 500,000	17%
Total Payer Receipts	**$3,000,000**	

In the above example you can see the payer with the highest dollar amount of charges is Cutten Mend Health at 50% of the total volume of charges. An analysis of your payer mix tells you more about your patient population.

Payer Productivity

In addition to the payer mix, we recommend running a payer productivity report regularly that ranks payers by receipts instead of charges. For example:

Table 17.5   Example Payer Productivity Report

Big Federal Insurance	$ 600,000	46%
Green Tea Health Plan	$ 500,000	39%
Cutten Mend Health	$ 200,000	15%
Total Payer Receipts	**$1,300,000**	

In the above example you can see that there is quite a difference between charges and receipts. There are several immediate takeaways: Big Federal has the highest dollar value of receipts even though the charges were lower; Green Tea Health is paying 100% of charges, which indicates the master fee schedule may be too low; and Cutten Mend Health, which represents 50% of our total charges is reimbursing at only 15% overall. This indicates that the provider's contract may be overdue for renegotiation.

Looking at data points across multiple reports will tell a story and you will be able to trend data across several dimensions to determine the true root cause of any issues. For example, if you take the above example and then look at an A/R aging report, you may identify that though Cutten Mend Health has very low receipts, they are more than 120 days behind in processing claims. If that's the case, you should review your payer contracts for timely payment clauses. Contact the insurance payer and request interest payments where applicable.

If you aren't sure where to find these reports, work with your practice management system vendor to locate or create them as needed.

✏ Chapter 17 Knowledge Check

Conducting an Internal Revenue Cycle Assessment

Question #1:

A profit and loss analysis should be reviewed _____ at minimum.

Question #2:

True or False? RVUs can be used as the foundation for provider compensation.

Question #3:

Circle One: Payer mix reports should be run by **charges** or **receipts**

Answers:

Q1: monthly,
Q2: True,
Q3: charges

Endnotes

1. https://www.healthit.gov/topic/privacy-security-and-hipaa/security-risk-assessment-tool
2. Book quote provided by: *Jay Hodes, President of Colington Consulting*
3. Book quote provided by: *Kathy Maddock, Maddock & Co.*

Chapter 18

Change Management

In larger industries, change management is something that's often discussed. For example, if you worked for an automobile manufacturing company and there was a significant change to the car manufacturing process, you would expect to see a structured set of change management processes. You would expect to see a document that defined the date the current process would end, the date to start using a new piece of equipment, how the new equipment works, how it is to be implemented, and perhaps an FAQ. You would anticipate training sessions with the team to discuss the changes and you would expect there to be full documentation summarizing all of this after the change was complete.

Hospitals often use change management processes. At the private practice level, especially in smaller practices, this is often not the case.

Change management involves supervising, navigating, and documenting all aspects of a significant change within your organization. If you aren't Six Sigma certified (a process improvement method) or familiar with DMAIC processes (define, measure, analyze, improve and control), don't panic. You can still take steps toward effective change management.

First, define the problem you need to solve, make sure to identify change leaders, and involve key participants. Document current processes, policies, and workflows and perform a Lean review. There is a lot that goes into a comprehensive lean review but focus on critical components like reducing duplication of effort.

Second, engage staff in the process of analyzing the problem and defining ways to improve. Once a solution is determined, provide education to all stakeholders and provide a platform for feedback. Implementing the solution isn't the end of your change process; it's really the middle. After implementation, you should still evaluate for ways to improve by scheduling look-back periods.

Third, provide for periods of internal and external auditing. Develop a process to limit repeated errors that are identified through the lookbacks and audits.

Finally, make sure you are educating all the stakeholders, which often extend beyond your practice.

For example, changes to your check-in process may leave patients feeling confused if they don't also receive some form of education on the change to the process that affects them.

Change Leaders

Whenever initiating significant change, the organization should identify change leaders. These are individuals who are not only excited for the change, but who are also ready to work with their boots to the ground to get the change implemented. Change leaders are invested in seeing the change all the way through and have the authority to support change implementation.

Key Participants

Key participants are those who must be at the table so the discussion will be comprehensive and include everyone involved in the process being changed. For example, a change in prior authorization processes means you probably need to include the billing department, the front desk, clinical staff, and perhaps, the Chief Medical Officer.

Critical components of the change can be missed when key participants are not at the table. For example, a change in prior office prior authorization processes may mean that the organization now needs to submit authorizations electronically. This may represent a change with who previously performed the prior authorization and with who needs access to the payer portal.

It's very likely that previously the only individuals who needed access to the payer portal were the front desk staff and the billing staff for the purposes of verifying eligibility, patient deductibles, etc. However, now that the prior authorization process is electronic, it is very likely the clinical department also needs access.

If the prior authorization process has changed due to a clinical reason, then the chief medical officer or supervising physician may want to be involved in that discussion. They may need to set new standing orders or parameters around the prior authorization process.

If any of these individuals are not at the table, then it's very possible the new authorization process implemented will not work as efficiently as intended.

Documentation

We all know the adage goes, "If you didn't document it, you didn't do it." For change management we modify that slightly to "If you didn't document it, it won't be done right."

One of the most impactful components of change management best practices is to document everything clearly and consistently. Use symbols within the organization in the same manner from process to process. Don't use a stop sign on one to mean "stop" when you want it to mean "go" on another.

There are three main benefits to documenting new processes: (1) documentation confirms that everyone's on the same page as far as the new processes are concerned, (2) it can be used as training material for staff, and (3) documenting the process also grants the practice the opportunity to perform a lean review.

Lean Review

The goal of a Lean review is to cut out unnecessary steps and reduce any duplication of effort. You may find during the documentation review that eligibility verification occurs three times. During the Lean review you can shift this task to the person with the most appropriate role and provide documentation that satisfies the needs of the other individuals who were previously performing the same task.

Steps of a Lean review:

1. Identify opportunities to reduce steps and duplication of efforts.

2. Create a plan for improvement.

3. Implement the plan/changes.

4. Look back to see how the changes have affected the overall outcomes and gain feedback from the team.

One of Lean's core principles is to set realistic targets or goals for performance improvement. Setting realistic goals encourages staff to stay motivated to achieve the desired target state. A best practice in setting realistic targets is to 'double the good or half the bad.' Simply put, let's say that your practice's goal is to collect a larger percentage of copayments at the time of service in order to reduce the time and cost of collecting that money owed following the date of service. The practice calculates that $10,000 of co-payments annually are currently not collected at the time of service. The practice, therefore, would set a target of reducing that number in half (or collecting $5,000 more annually). This goal setting principal can be applied to various components of the RCM process, including aging account receivables, charge entry lag, clean claim processing, etc.[1]

Brian Ramos, MBA, CMPE, Chief Operating Officer of Capital Anesthesia Partners

Staff Engagement

Change management should also include engaging staff. Staff need to be excited about and involved in the change for it to be effective. When individuals are engaged in the process and become part of the change, it strengthens the impact of the overall change. Individuals who feel the weight of their role in the organization are more likely to perform at a meets or exceeds expectations level.

Education and Feedback

Employees need to know exactly what they're changing and the impetus behind it. They need to have knowledge of business processes, and they need to understand when and how to escalate issues or concerns.

A platform for feedback is also important because it provides a method for continuous improvement. For every new process implemented there should be a look-back period. Typically, this is about 90 days after the change has gone into effect. This gives everyone involved enough time to work out the kinks, for the staff to be trained, and for the processes to be incorporated into the business.

If after 90 days everything is running smoothly then you know that the process you used to educate and engage your staff is a good one and you can continue to use. If, however, and this is more likely, there were a few bumps along the way, then this gives you the opportunity to look at those errors to prevent them from occurring in the future.

Auditing (Internal & External)

Internal and external auditing is also a way to review change management processes. This is more common in much larger institutions, but regardless of the size of the organization it would be beneficial in any highly regulated facility. For example, let's say you have an onsite pharmacy that regularly dispenses controlled substances and you're beginning to change workflow processes related to inventory controls. It may be beneficial to perform an external and internal audit to confirm that the new processes comply with federal and state regulations.

Voluntary audits can identify areas of weakness in processes and can highlight potential compliance concerns.

Patient Education

Patient education is also part of the change management process. Remember, patients see more than we think they do. If patients call in quarterly to have a medication prescription authorized for refill, then they're used to speaking with the same person each time. If suddenly this process changes and patients are unaware of it, then staff should educate patients of this change and assure them they will still be able to get the authorization they need.

Communicating process changes at the practice with patients can be completed over the phone, in a letter, on the practice website, or as part of the phone tree when patients dial in. The main objective is to interact with patients and prevent frustration, especially when patients inquire about changes.

✏ Chapter 18 Knowledge Check

Change Management

Question #1:

True or False? Making a process Lean means removing unnecessary steps and duplication of effort.

Question #2:

True or False? Key participants for change only include the practice owner.

Question #3:

True or False? A look-back period should be performed after a large change has been implemented to look for improvement opportunities.

Answer:

Q1: True,
Q2: False,
Q3: True

Endnotes

1. Book quote provided by: *Brian Ramos, MBA, CMPE, Chief Operating Officer of Capital Anesthesia Partners*

APPENDICES

Appendix A

Patient Demographics

Patient demographics refer to the individual data required to create a profile for the patient.[1] Obtaining and maintaining accurate patient demographic data is a critical component of revenue cycle management as well as operational and financial management process. Patient demographic fields include the following:

Patient Identifiers	First Name, Middle Name, Last Name, Prefixes/Suffixes, Date of Birth, Race, Ethnicity, Social Security Number, Internal Account Numbers or Patient Identifiers, Driver's License (Number and Image), Headshot photo, Primary Language, Marital Status, Status of Citizenship (where required)
	For Pediatrics: Include Parent's Names, Contact Information, Custody/Legal Agreements as needed
Patient Contact Information	Phone Numbers (Work, Cell/Mobile, Home), Email Address, Home Address, Business Address
Patient Emergency Contacts	Name, Address, Relationship, Phone, and Email of Emergency Contacts, Scope of Information Permitted to Release
Accessibility and Assistance	Needs for: Hearing, Transportation, Vision, Ambulation, Language, Interpreters, or other assistance either needed or in place

---

[1] https://www.himssinnovationcenter.org/immunization-integration-program/data-elements-for-patient-demographics

Insurance Information	Insurance Carrier, Payer Number, Plan Name, Plan Number, Group Number, RX BIN Number, Subscriber ID Number, Subscriber Name, Subscriber Date of Birth, Subscriber Social Security Number, Claims Submission Address, Full Copy of Front and Back of Card, Amounts if listed (copay, coinsurance, deductible), Insurer Phone Number,
Care Team	Patient's Primary Care Provider, Specialty Providers, Preferred Pharmacy, Caregivers (including home health or hospice care)
Financial Information	Guarantor on Account, Guarantor's Relationship, Guarantor's Phone Numbers (Work, Cell/Mobile, Home), Guarantor's Email Address, Guarantor's Home Address
Legal Notices	Filed Power of Attorney, Filed Do Not Resuscitate, Any other legal notifications required or beneficial

Appendix B

Provider Credentialing Questionnaire

The Provider Credentialing Questionnaire is a useful tool for collecting and maintaining critical demographic data from your providers. Credentialing is an ongoing process and even if your practice uses a system like CAQH (Council for Affordable Quality Healthcare) you should retain this information in a provider file for permanent reference. Unfortunately, not all providers will be a lifer at your organization which means you may one day lose access to their CAQH profile. This template can aid you in capturing key pieces of information.

First Name:_____ Middle_____ Last Name _____ Credential: _____

Alias/DBA/Other Names: _____

Place of Birth _____ Date of Birth _____/_____/_____

SSN _____ Tax ID _____

Practice Location _____

Pay to Address _____

Billing Address _____

Home Address _____

Business Phone _____ Fax# _____

Cell _____ Business Email:_____

Personal Email _____ Provider NPI# _____

Group NPI# _____

Driver's License _____ Issuing State __ Expiration Date _____

DEA# _____Expiration Date _____

CDS# _____ Expiration Date _____

Board Certification(s): _____

License# _____ Issuing State _____ Expiration Date _____

License# _____ Issuing State _____ Expiration Date _____

Medical School _____ Attendance _____ To _____

Medical School _____ Attendance _____ To _____

Practice Information

Office Hours Mon ____Tues ____Wed ____Thurs ____Fri _____

After Hours Coverage _____EHR/PM Software Vendor _____

Number and type of providers in your practice: _____

Practice Website: _____ Practice Email: _____

Payer Participation

PECOS Authorized Official _____ User ID _____ Password _____

CAQH User ID _____ Password _____

Medicaid Username _____ Password _____

Medicare Participation Yes _____No ____PTAN# _____State _____

Medicaid Participation Yes _____No ____State _____State _____

<u>Top 5 Target Payers for Participation</u>

Payer Effective Date Renewal Date Group or Individual Participation

_____

_____

_____

_____

Please provide current copies of the following documents:

- Board Certificate
- DEA
- CDS
- Medical License
- Curriculum Vitae
- Fellowship, Residency, and Diploma
- Malpractice Certificate
- 5 years of malpractice claims history and license/hospital sanctions
- Letter from bank with routing and account numbers for EFTs
- Voided check
- W-9
- IRS CP-575 Form (for Medicare enrollment)
- DUNS #
- State Department of Assessment & Taxation SDAT#
- CLIA Certificate (for Medicare and MD Medicaid enrollment)
- Lab and X-ray Certificate if applicable (for MD Medicaid enrollment)
- Delegation Agreement for applicable non-physician providers

Appendix C

Preliminary RCM Questionnaire

The following is a Preliminary RCM Questionnaire, your billing manager should be able to fill this form with ease. This is useful for new managers gaining familiarity, for discovery during mergers and acquisitions, or for consultants looking to obtain baseline RCM demographics for an organization.

1. Number of providers _____ Types _____ Taxonomy Codes _____

2. EHR/PM Software: Clearinghouse:

3. In-House or Outsourced Billing:

4. Average totals for: Unique Pt Visits Charges Payments Adjustments Credit Bal.

   a. Daily

   b. Monthly

   c. Annually

5. What is the payer mix (i.e., percentage of Medicare, Medicaid, and BCBS)?

   a. Payer 1 _____   % of volume _____

   b. Payer 2 _____   % of volume _____

   c. Payer 3 _____   % of volume _____

    d. Payer 4_____ % of volume _____

    e. Payer 5_____ % of volume _____

6. Aging A/R Dollars:

    30 Days _____ 45 Days _____ 60 Days _____

    90 Days _____ 120 Days _____

7. Annual Collections per TIN: Annual Charges per TIN:

8. Participation in Incentive programs:

9. Frequency of processing refunds:

10. Frequency of sending patient statements: _____ Methods used: _____

11. Accepted forms of payment from patients:

    ❑ Patient Portal ❑ Credit ❑ Checks ❑ Cash

12. Accept insurance company EFT's: Yes or No Payer Credit Cards: Yes or No

13. Methods used for insurance verification:

14. Contingency fee charged by bad debt collections agency:

15. Monthly dollar amount sent to bad debt:

16. Average monthly bad debt agency collections:

17. Average daily patient volumes:

18. In-patient Hospital services performed: ❑ Yes or ❑ No Number of hospitals: _____

19. Date of last charge master review and charge amount increase:

20. Date of last fee schedule analysis:

21. Date of last managed care contract review and negotiation:

22. Date of last internal coding review:

Appendix D

Front Office Operations

As we've covered in this book, the front office is critical to the success of any revenue cycle model. Therefore, it is essential to assess the performance and education of your front desk operations on a regular basis. The following assessment should be used as a starting point for your assessments.

It may behoove you to include additional topics for assessment and we encourage you to do so. During your assessment, be on the lookout for issues which may impact revenue, compliance, or otherwise cause risk for the organization.

Practice Area	Assessment
Daily Patient Volumes	
Patient Satisfaction	
Superbill/charge master review	
Badge ID	
Front Desk Documents review	
Patient Arrival & Sign In	
Auth/Referral/Pre-cert Process	
Cross Training to cover multiple roles	

Appointment Confirmation	
End of Day Reconciliation	
Internal Controls	
Petty Cash for Patient Transactions	
Insurance Verification	
Daily Staffing Levels	
Scheduling	
Medical Records Requests	
Medical Record Copying Fees	
Faxing and Scanning	
Work Space	
Check-In	
Intake forms	
Notice of Privacy Practices	
Check-Out	
Merchant Services	
Call Center	
Parking	
EHR Inbox	
Staff Appearance and Identification	

Appendix E

Billing, Collections, & Coding

Like the front desk assessment, the billing, collections, and coding assessment is a key component in successfully diagnosing existing or potential risks to your revenue cycle model.

The following assessment should be used as a starting point for your assessments. It may behoove you to include additional topics for assessment and we encourage you to do so. During your assessment, be on the lookout for issues which may impact revenue, compliance, or otherwise cause risk for the organization.

Practice Area	Assessment
Charge Entry	
Medicare Secondary Payer (MSP) Forms	
Advanced Beneficiary Notice (ABN)	
Code Selection / EHR Encoding	
SNOMED or GEMS via EHR	
Documentation Guidelines 1995 or 1997	
Code Books and Resources	
Coding Audits	
Claim Submission	

Clearinghouse	
Claims Edit Report Resolution	
A/R Follow Up Process	
Payer A/R Assignments	
EOM Report Packages	
Incentive Program Participation: MIPS Status	
Service Reconciliation	
Cash/Daily Collections Reconciliations	
Appeals process	
Recovery Auditor Contractor (RAC) Responses	
Payer Trend Denials	
Payer mix	
Patient A/R – Patient Statements	
Bad Debt	
A/R Reports -Referring Physician -Business Recap -Adjustment/Write-Off -Credit Balance -Aging A/R & Bad Debt -Company History Analysis -Payer Mix -Schedule Status Analysis -Active Patients -Productivity & Profitability -Site, Provider, CPT, Payer	

Adjustments and Write-Offs	
Payment Posting and Deposits	
Fee Schedule Analysis	
Charge Master	
EFT/ERA	
Insurance Refunds/Retractions	
Patient Refunds	
Patient Account Balance Review Prior to Visit	
Virtual Payments	
Billing Staff Performance Monitoring	
Billing Company Scope of Work	
Billing Company Contract on file	
Credit Balances	

Appendix F

Internal Refund Request Form

Practice Header

REFUND REQUEST

Date:	Amount to Refund: $
Detailed Reason for Refund:	

Issue Refund Payable to:

Address to Mail Refund to:

Refund will not be processed without the following items completed:

- ❏ Supporting Document Attached
- ❏ Documentation in PM system

Employee Submitting to Finance:

Date Received by Finance: _____ Date Approved:_____

Refund Amount Issued:

Check/ACH Number:

Date of Issuance:

_____   _____

Printed Name of Person Approving Refund   Signature of Person Approving Refund

Appendix G

Financial Hardship Application

Patient Name: _____ Date: _____

Patient Address:_____

Request for financial hardship is based upon:

❏ Homelessness   ❏ Income/Employment   ❏ Natural Disaster   ❏ Bankruptcy

❏ Other: _____

Employment Status: ❏ Unemployed   ❏ Retired   ❏ Disabled   ❏ Employed _____ hrs/wk

Primary Insurance Information:

Plan _____ Effective Date: _____

ID# _____ Subscriber: _____

SSN _____

Secondary Insurance Information:

Plan _____ Effective Date:_____

ID# _____ Subscriber:_____

SSN _____

Supporting Information

# of Dependents in the home _____ Weekly Income_____

Have supporting documents been attached?   ❏ Yes   ❏ No

Other Comments:_____

_____

_____

_____

_____

I _____ (patient/guarantor) hereby certify that the above documented information is true to the best of my knowledge. I further confirm that should a significant change in financial hardship occur, I will notify the practice and revise this application.

_____   _____

Patient's Signature   Date

Appendix H

Electronic Health Record (EHR) Compatibility

Use this EHR compatibility reminder list as a resource when vetting software for your practice

- CCHIT Certification
- Stand out features
- References from practices in your specialty and in your market
- Implementation process support
- Customer service/support
- Comparison to other software competition
- Provider/Practice turn-over rate
- Number of current client practices/providers
- Highest geographic market
- Highest specialty practice market
- HIE interfacing
- All fees (licensing, implementation, training, transactions, RCM, maintenance)
- Interfacing capabilities (labs, radiology)
- Diagnosis code look up
- Procedure code and modifier selection
- ICD-10-CM code tool (SNOMED, GEMS, etc.)

- Coding convention being used 1995 or 1997
- Template customization (CCM, TCM, smart phrases, physician notes, transcription interfaces)
- Date and sources of annual coding updates
- Clearinghouse interface
- Back up: Frequency, disaster plan and data retrieval
- RCM capabilities
- Merchant Services interface capabilities and cost
- Average percent of patients utilizing patient portal
- Online payment capability
- Popular financial reports
- Eligibility check capabilities and transaction fees
- Digital office automation (eFax set, scanning, internal communications)
- Medication Management
- Pharmacy interface – ePrescribing & electronic prescribing of controlled substances (EPCS)
- Patient portal
- Server-based technology or cloud-based
- Open API
- Telehealth technology
- Exit strategy
  - ○ Perpetual access to current software
  - ○ Data migration formats and turnaround time
- PM software interface capabilities

Appendix I

Checklist

Recommended Competency Standards for Staff Performing Verifications

- Counsel patients on the details of their insurance benefits and referral obligations.

- Perform insurance verifications and pre-authorizations on required services. Verify and obtain all eligibilities and referral requirements prior to services being rendered.

- Document all eligibility and referral requirements for use during registration/intake. Update patient account and superbill with new information received during eligibility checks. Assist in obtaining referrals from referring physicians as needed.

- Call patients to confirm appointments and notify them of referral requirements and insurance eligibility.

- Review and correct billing and referral forms, checking for accuracy and completeness before data entry.

- Coordinate, schedule, and pre-authorize diagnostic testing with offsite facilities. Counsel patients on testing location, time, insurance guidelines, and pre-op instructions.

- Complete accurate verbal pre-registration prior to patient's appointments. Obtain and accurately document patient demographic, clinical, and insurance information.

- Make sure patient appointments and physician schedules are prepared in an accurate manner.

- Adhere to contracted payer reimbursement guidelines and federal and state regulations related to HIPAA security and patient privacy compliance.

- Use professional telephone etiquette, take accurate messages, and relay those messages in a timely manner. Review patient accounts and notify patients of any balances.

- Accurately scan and file medical records in electronic format. Ensure scanning does not become backlogged throughout the day. Double-check that records contain appropriate information.

- Assist with check-in and check-out functions as needed to include registration and balance collection.

Glossary

Word	Definition	Acronym (where applicable)
Abuse	Abuse describes practices that, either directly or indirectly, result in unnecessary costs to the Medicare Program. Abuse includes any practice inconsistent with providing patients with medically necessary services meeting professionally recognized standards.	Included in FWA, as the "A"
Account Number (Medical Record Number)	Unique number assigned to securely identify each patient in EHR/PM software. This number is used internally by the practice to identify the patient.	
Accountable Care Organization	ACOs are groups of doctors, hospitals, and other health care providers, who come together voluntarily for the purposes of providing coordinated care for the purposes of better health outcomes, decreased cost of care and distribution of cost savings from Medicare.	ACO
Accounts Receivable	Amounts in A/R are outstanding balances due payable to the organization. This can include balances due from patients as well as from insurers.	A/R

Advanced Beneficiary Notice	An ABN is a letter officially informing you that your healthcare provider or supplier believes that Medicare will not cover an item(s) and/or service(s). The ABN helps you make an informed choice about whether or not you want to receive the item(s) and/or service(s) knowing that you may be responsible for payment. Remember, if you decide to receive the item(s) and/or services, you may be financially responsible for those charges.	ABN
Advance Care Planning	Face-to-face service between a physician (or other qualified health care professional) and a patient discussing advance directives with or without completing relevant legal forms. This service is paid by Medicare separately or as an element of an AWV.	
Alternative Payment Models	An APM is a payment approach that gives added incentive payments to provide high-quality and cost-efficient care. APMs can apply to a specific clinical condition, a care episode, or a population.	APMs
Allowed Amount	The maximum contracted amount that is paid by a health insurance company for a covered service. Other terms used are: Negotiated rate, eligible expense and payment allowance. Participation agreements typically required a healthcare provider, to accept this payment amount in full.	
Ambulatory Care	Healthcare services provided on an out-patient basis at a medical office or Ambulatory Surgical Center.	
Ambulatory Payment Classification	A unit of payment most frequently used in the hospital OPPS (outpatient prospective payment system)	APC

Ambulatory Surgery Center	An outpatient surgery center where less complicated procedures can be performed as long as they don't require an overnight stay.	ASC
Annual Wellness Visit	A preventative wellness service that includes a health risk assessment and personalize prevention plan. There is no cost to eligible Medicare beneficiaries.	AWV
Anti-Kickback Statute	The AKS is a criminal law that prohibits the knowing and willful payment of remuneration to induce or reward patient referrals or the generation of business involving any item or service payable by the federal health care programs (e.g., drugs, supplies, or healthcare services for Medicare or Medicaid patients).	AKS
Antitrust Laws	Overseen by the Department of Justice, these laws prevent anticompetitive conduct which in turn helps to contain healthcare costs, improve quality, provide choices for patients and foster healthcare innovation.	
Appeal	A healthcare provider may disagree with the claims adjudication or decision by a health plan. Depending upon the insurance company, there are a number of methods in which a provider may request a review and reconsideration of the manner in which a claim was or was not paid.	
Assignment of Benefits	AOB occurs when one provider wants the payment for their services sent elsewhere. For example, an employed provider in a group practice may reassign their individual benefits to the group practice for collection and posting.	AOB

Authorized Official	A legal representative of a medical practice or healthcare organization. This individual has authority to sign and enroll the organization into Medicare or other health plans. This individual may assign permission to other individuals within the organization to perform tasks on behalf of the organization. Examples are President, Physician Owner, or CEO.
Bad Debt	This generally refers to an amount that has been sent to collections or an amount that has been difficult to collect from the patient.
Balance Billing	Occurs when a healthcare provider charges/bills a patient for balance between the provider's charge amount which was billed to insurance and the allowed amount; which, for participating providers is the contract rate. Participating providers are not permitted to balance bill patients.
Benchmarking	Process of comparing and measuring areas of your practice with industry best practices and standards.
Beneficiary	Individual who is covered by health plan benefits. The health plan has contractually agreed to pay for certain covered services for this individual.
Birthday Rule	Used for coordination of insurance benefits for children whose parents have separate health insurance plans. The insurance for the parent whose birthday is earlier in the year than the other will be listed as the primary insurance. In the event the parents birthdays are on the same day, the insurance plan that provided coverage the longest will be primary.

Bundled Service	These are services that have been grouped together during a certain timeframe for payment purposes. Any codes in the same bundle cannot be billed or reimbursed separately. This is common when one procedure always requires another.	
Capitation	This is a payment arrangement in which the provider is paid a flat amount for each patient they have attributed or for each patient they have enrolled. In capitated arrangements, the provider will receive the same payment whether the patient is seen twice or fifteen times.	
Carve Outs	This refers to specific codes on negotiated fee schedules for which separate reimbursement methodologies have been made. It is common to have a straight percentage of increase across the board. However, a practice may want a higher rate on a few more frequent procedures. This would be an example of a carve out.	
Centers for Medicare and Medicaid Services	The federal agency within the Department of Health and Human Services (HHS) that administers the Medicare program. Among its responsibilities, CMS oversees the Medicare Administrative Contractors involved in the processing and review of Medicare claims at the first and second level of appeals.	CMS
Central Billing Office	A central billing office dedicates staff to billing tasks without giving them alternate responsibilities. The goal is to have a centralized team with one singular focus for the improvement of billing processes and workflows.	CBO

Charge Description Master	List of CPT® codes and HCPCS and descriptions of the services a practice performs on its patients. The listed amount that a practice charges for each service is included. This list should be reviewed and updated regularly.	CDM
Charge Entry/ Capture	The data entry of services performed along with their charge amount from the fee schedule so that a claim can be billed to the insurance company.	
Children's Health Insurance Program	Insurance program that provides low-cost health coverage to children in families that earn too much money to qualify for Medicaid but not enough to buy private insurance. In some states, CHIP covers pregnant women.	CHIP
Chronic Care Management	Each state offers CHIP coverage and works closely with its state Medicaid program.	CCM
Claim	A claim is a request to the insurance company for payment for items and services rendered by the provider to a patient.	
Claim Adjustment Reason Codes	Communicate an adjustment, meaning that they must communicate why a claim or service line was paid differently than it was billed.	CARC
Claim Control Number	The CCN is an individual 14-digit number given to each claim when entered into the Medicare system. The first five digits indicate the date (in Julian date format) Medicare received the claim. The Julian date will equal the first two digits of the year and the next three digits are the sequential numbering of the days of the year (March 23, 2007 will show 07083). The sixth digit indicates whether the claim was submitted electronically or paper. The final digit indicates whether the claim is an initial or adjusted claim. A final number of 1 or higher shows the claim has been adjusted.	CCN

Claim Submission	The act of submitting a medical services claim to the insurance company for payment.
Clean Claims Act	State specific law requiring insurance companies to pay claims to provider that have no errors or incomplete documentation in a specified amount of time.
Clearinghouse	This is the intermediary between the practice and the insurance company. Typically practices submit claims to insurances through the clearinghouse which performs a review for errors before submitting to the insurance company. The clearinghouse also has eligibility check capabilities and bi-directional Practice Management software interface.
Clinically Laboratory Improvement Amendments	A certification for labs which validates quality laboratory practices. CLIA certification is required to receive laboratory service payments from Medicare and Medicaid.	CLIA
Clinically Integrated Network	A group of providers, practices, and/or hospitals which joined together to support cost reduction through collaboration. These groups target commercial payers and do not solely focus on Medicare shared savings. Tax ID#'s participating in a CIN that meet federal guidelines may be exempt from anti-trust/kick-back laws.	CIN
Cloning	This is a term commonly used to refer to using copy and paste, or templates, to fill the majority of the patient's encounter note.
Code Set 270	Secure file format used by providers to query medical benefits to a patients insurance.
Code Set 271	Secure file format sent back from a patients insurance that provides medical benefits for their beneficiary.
Code Set 835	Secure file format used for payment or electronic remittance advice from an insurance company to a provider.

Code Set 837	Secure file format used to electronically submit health insurance claims.	
Co-insurance	The remaining balance for a covered service that is the patient's responsibility to pay after a deductible has been met. A calculation example is: Insurance pays 80% and leaves 20% as a co-insurance/patient responsibility.	
Co-payment	A flat-rate that a patient would pay to a healthcare provider for covered services. There are varying tiers of co-payment amounts such as: Primary Care, Specialist, Urgent Care, Emergency Room, and Pharmacy. This amount is determined by the insurer. Patients are notified of this amount during the insurance enrollment process or it is indicated on their insurance card. The provider is informed through their insurance participation agreement to collect this amount from the patient. Healthcare providers are advised to collect co-payments at the time service is rendered.	
Collections	This term can have two meanings: 1) the receipts/revenue collected during a specific timeframe 2) A/R sent to a collections agency as bad debt	
Collections Ratio	This number reflects the days in A/R or in other words the number of days it takes the company to convert A/R into receipts.	
Commercial Health Insurance	An insurance plan that is not funded by a government entity.	
Comprehensive Error Rate Testing	The CERT program measures payment compliance with Medicare FFS program federal rules, regulations, and requirements	CERT

Consolidated Omnibus Reconciliation Act	The Consolidated Omnibus Budget Reconciliation Act (COBRA) gives workers and their families who lose their health benefits the right to choose to continue group health benefits provided by their group health plan for limited periods of time under certain circumstances such as voluntary or involuntary job loss, reduction in the hours worked, transition between jobs, death, divorce, and other life events.	COBRA
Consultation	A meeting with a professional or subject matter expert to better understand a specific situation, idea, or program.	
Consumer Assessment of Healthcare Providers and Systems	The Consumer Assessment of Healthcare Providers and Systems (CAHPS) is a series of patient surveys and assessments that help assess the quality of patient experience. These surveys are overseen by the Agency for Healthcare Research and Quality (AHRQ).	CAHPS
Contractual Allowance	This refers to the amount that is allowed by the contract per the negotiated fee schedule.	
Conversion Factor	This is the base number that Medicare uses to generate fees per RVU. Geographic Adjustment Factors (GAFs) are often applied to this number to account for regional variations in cost.	CF
Coordination of Benefits	If a beneficiary has more than one insurance, COB rules decide which entity pays first.	COB
Cost Sharing	The portion of healthcare costs that a patient pays out of pocket that are not covered by their insurance plan.	
Credentialing	The process by which provider information is provided and updated with the insurance payers and accuracy is confirmed for provider enrollment and participation.	

Credit Balance	When an overpayment has occurred resulting in the practice having received more money than what was due for a particular account.	
Cross-File	This is the process by which claims are submitted to the next payer responsible. For example, a primary payer sending a copy of their EOB to the secondary payer on file.	
Current Procedural Terminology	CPT® codes are the United States' standard for how medical professionals document and report medical, surgical, radiology, laboratory, anesthesiology, and evaluation and management (E/M) services. All healthcare providers, payers, and facilities use CPT® codes. The five-character CPT® codes are used by insurers to help determine the amount of reimbursement that a practitioner will receive for services provided.	CPT
Date of Service	The date in which healthcare services were rendered by a healthcare provider to a patient.	DOS
Days in Accounts Receivable	The number of days an outstanding claim balance has been on the books without full resolution.	
Deductible	In addition to monthly premiums, some health plans have an additional expense that patients must pay to activate payment for healthcare services. An insurance company will not begin paying for services until the applicable deductible is met. Once met, the patient's co-insurance would apply.	
Delegated Official	This means an individual who is delegated by the "Authorized Official," the authority to report changes and updates to the enrollment record. The delegated official must be an individual with an ownership or control interest in (as that term is defined in section 1124(a)(3) of the Social Security Act), or be a W-2 managing employee of, the provider or supplier.	

Denial	Decision not to authorize payments or services or supplies.	
Dependents	Individuals who are covered by an insurance plan of which they are not the subscriber.	
Diagnosis Code	This refers to the classification of condition or ailment by code. The current classification used in the US is ICD-10	
Diagnosis Related Group	DRGs are a patient classification scheme which provides a means of relating the type of patients a hospital treats (i.e., its case mix) to the costs incurred by the hospital.	DRG
Distant Site	Location of the eligible health care provider who is performing telehealth services.	
Dual Eligible	Beneficiaries who are eligible for both Medicare Part A and or Part B and Medicaid benefits.	
Duplicate Claim	When a claim for the same patient, DOS, and procedures is submitted more than once to the same insurer, it is listed as a duplicate claim because the original has already been submitted.	
Durable Medical Equipment	This is equipment which is medically needed for the benefit of sick or disabled patients. Example: Walkers, Blood Sugar Monitor, Oxygen Equipment, etc.	DME
Elective Services	Healthcare services that are found to be medically appropriate by the provider and patient but may not be covered by the patient's insurance plan. These services are planned and not emergent such as cosmetic surgery and fertility treatments.	
Electronic Data Interchange	Secure exchange of healthcare data amongst healthcare institutions, health insurance and providers. It is also used for claims processing.	EDI
Electronic Funds Transfer	The transference of funds electronically from one party to another, typically directly from bank account to bank account	EFT

Electronic Medical Record	An electronically maintained record of the patients medical information.	EMR
Electronic Remittance Advice	An electronic version of the EOB. This document explains the payments, adjustments, and denials processed for a given number of claims.	ERA
Eligibility Identification Management	This is the process by which individuals, businesses, and third parties can apply for and receive a single User ID they may be used to securely access many CMS applications.	EIDM
Eligibility Verification System or Electronic Visit Verification	This system is access to healthcare providers for the purposes of confirming a patients state Medicaid benefits eligibility which may be performed electronically or by telephone. Many electronic systems will indicate the name of the applicable Medicaid Managed Care Organization (MCO) that a beneficiary may be assigned.	EVS or EVV
Encounter	This refers to the instances of patient interactions whether the patient is on-site or remote. This term is often used synonymously with "visit"	
Enroll	The process to request participation and eligibility to submit claims to health plans.	
Episode of Care	Services provided to treat a clinical condition or procedure within a set time period.	
Established Patient	An established patient is one who has received professional services from the physician/qualified health care professional or another physician/ qualified health care professional of the exact same specialty and subspecialty who belongs to the same group practice, within the past three years.	

Evaluation and Management	A category of CPT ® codes used for identifying services provided and translating those services into billable codes used for reimbursement. These codes vary based on service complexity and specific documentation requirements. There are two guidelines for E&M services: 1995 and 1997. Providers should not combine 1995 and 1997 within the same encounter. The overarching variance between the two guidelines is the documentation of the examination performed within a visit. Specialists who are focused on a certain body system, tend to favor the use of 1997 guidelines. The 1995 guidelines however, allow for more flexibility by stating that 2-7 body systems were addressed and documented.	E&M
Excluded Services	This refers to services that are not covered by the insurer.	
Explanation of Benefits	This is a summary of services provided, payments made, non-payments or denials, adjustments allocated and patient responsibilities owed. This is a paper document mailed to the provider by the insurance plan.	EOB
False Claims Act	This Federal law states that anyone who has knowingly submitted false healthcare claims for the purposes of defrauding the government is liable to be penalized. The statute provides that one who is liable must pay a civil penalty.	
Federal Register	This is the official documentation repository for the federal government. All public notices, proposed rules and agency regulations are posted here daily.	

Federally Qualified Healthcare Center	Community-based health care providers that receive funds from the HRSA Health Center Program to provide primary care services in underserved areas. They must meet a stringent set of requirements, including providing care on a sliding fee scale based on ability to pay and operating under a governing board that includes patients.	FQHC
Fee for Service	Payment for healthcare services and supplies individually by Medicare.	FFS
Fee Schedule	A fee schedule is a complete listing of payments made by a payer to reimburse providers and suppliers.	
Financial Hardship	Occasionally, payment of copays, deductibles and other patient responsibilities will cause undue strain on the patient. In these cases patients are assessed for "financial hardship" to determine if the patient qualifies for an exemption which would absolve them of these responsibilities.	
Financial Policy	A notice provided to patients regarding a practice's policies related to financial matters concerning healthcare services and administrative operations. This notice may include a patient's financial responsibilities and the manner in which a practice intends on billing for services and supplies.	
Fraud	Medicare fraud typically includes any of the following: ● Knowingly submitting, or causing to be submitted, false claims or making misrepresentations of fact to obtain a Federal health care payment for which no entitlement would otherwise exist	Included in FWA as the F

- Knowingly soliciting, receiving, offering, and/or paying remuneration to induce or reward referrals for items or services reimbursed by Federal health care programs

- Making prohibited referrals for certain designated health services

Fraud Waste and Abuse	This stands for Fraud, Waste, and Abuse	FWA
Geographic Practice Cost Index	An adjustment factor used to accommodate for regional variations in costs for providing care in different geographic locations. This factor is used to reallocate payment rates to reflect variations in regional practice expenses.	GPCI
Global Payment	Some services require a period of monitoring afterward. Any services rendered the period thereafter are bundled into the initial payment. This is referred to as a global payment of services.	
Glossary	This glossary is a compilation of terms used in health care reimbursement, insurance benefits and related medical terminology.	
Gross Charges	This is the total amount of charges billed for a particular date of service.	
Guarantor	This is the term used for the person responsible for making payments on a patient's account. For example, on a pediatric account, one of their parents would like be the guarantor.	
Health Insurance	This type of insurance covers patients for certain health services in return for a scheduled prepayment of premiums.	
Health Care Financing Administration 1500 Form	A form previously used to submit paper healthcare services to insurance plans for reimbursement.	HCFA

Health Insurance Portability & Accountability Act	Federal regulation that covered entities are required to provide safeguards for the privacy and security of protected health information that is created, stored, transmitted and received by the entity. This law includes a privacy and security act. The law provides patients certain rights over their health information including rights to examine and obtain a copy of their health records, and to request corrects.	HIPAA
Health Maintenance Organization	An entity that pays for healthcare services to beneficiaries who use their pre-approved network of providers and healthcare facilities. Use of providers outside of the network may result in higher out of pocket expenses to a beneficiary. Some HMOs require patient to obtain a referral to see a specialist.	HMO
Health Plan Employer Data and Information Set	Measures used to track performance of health plans. This data is pulled from healthcare providers, benchmarked and reported to which then rates health plans based on a scoring system. NCQA also uses this information for health plan accreditation. This information is also used by health plans to make improvements where needed.	HEDIS
Health Reimbursement Account	Funds allocated by an employer paid to an employee for the reimbursement of out of pocket healthcare expenses which may personal insurance premiums. This arrangement yields tax advantages for both the employer and the employee.	HRA
Healthcare Common Procedural Coding System Level II	A standardized coding system that is used primarily to identify products, supplies, and services not included in the CPT codes, such as ambulance services and durable medical equipment, prosthetics, orthotics, and supplies (DMEPOS) when used outside a physician's office.	HCPCS

Hierarchical Condition Categories	Risk-adjustment model used to estimate future healthcare costs. ICD-10 codes are mapped to these categories and risk scores are assigned to patients. Other factors such as age, gender and other demographics are included in the risk score. A risk adjustment factor (RAF) is used to predict healthcare costs. The two types of HCCs are CMS and HHS. HCCs may be reported at least once a calendar year.	HCC
ICD-10-CM	International Statistical Classification of Diseases and Health Related Problems, 10th revision developed a clinical modification of the classification for morbidity purposes. Used to code and classify diagnoses, symptoms, injury, abnormal findings, and external causes. This code set allows for enhanced specificity by including location, severity, cause and manifestation.	ICD-10
In-network	A healthcare provider is enrolled and participating in a health insurance panel and has the ability to receive reimbursement at a rate only offered to paneled providers.	
Incident To	Services that are provided by a qualified non-physician practitioner in a qualified out-patient setting but billed under an eligible physician's provider or NPI. These services are paid at 100% of the allowable amount.	
Insurance Verification	The process of confirming insurance coverage for a patient. This process should be done prior to services or supplies being rendered. This confirmation process includes a provider representative making contact with the patients insurance plan to confirm information to include but not limited to copay, deductible, effective date, benefits for services, and claims address.	

The Joint Commission	An independent non-profit organization that accredits and certifies healthcare organizations and programs with a nationally recognized accreditation. Accredited organizations must meet certain performance standards.	The Joint Commission or TJC
Jurisdiction Locality	Geographic region serviced by a Medicare MAC.	
Key Performance Indicator	Measurable value used to determine the success of pre-determined goals and objectives. Development of these indicators should include extractable data, comparisons to be measured in a variety of ways. Examples of KPIs are CPT productivity, reimbursement by payer, provider productivity. Data should be used for improvements and decision making.	KPI
Local Coverage Determinations	A service coverage determination that is authorized to be made by a Medicare MAC for services or items that are reasonable and necessary. The MAC makes an LCD when there is no NCD guidance or if NCD guidance requires further clarity in a particular region.	LCD
Managed Care Organization	Contracted agreement between an health services organization with a state Medicaid agency for the purposes of providing healthcare benefits and other services to Medicaid beneficiaries. MCO's are also tasked with managing quality, utilization and cost.	MCO
Meaningful Use	A government quality-program designed to penalize low-performing providers and bonus high-performing providers based upon successful achievement of specific quality metrics commonly referred to as CQMs (clinical quality measures). This program has been phased out.	MU

Medicaid	State and Federally funded health insurance for low income individuals.	
Medically Unlikely Edits	CMS created claims edits to reduce the error rate for payment of Part B claims. The three sets of edits are DME, facility and practitioners. CMS will deny payment for services that exceed the maximum units of service a provider would normally report for a beneficiary on a date of service.	MUE
Medicare	A federal health insurance program that primarily covers individuals age 65 or older who have contributed to the Medicare system during their lifetime. Medicare provides coverage for annual prevention services, sick visits, and hospital visits. Some plans therein also include DME and prescriptions.	Mcare
Medicare Access and Chip Reauthorization Act	Bipartisan legislation created the Quality Payment Program (QPP) which repeals the Sustainable Growth Rate (SGR) formula, rewards clinicians for quality over volume, combines multiple programs under the MIPS and gives bonus payments for participation in APMs.	MACRA
Medicare Advantage Plan (Part C)	Health benefits coverage offered under a policy or contract by an MS organization that includes a specific set of health benefits offered at a uniform premium and uniform level of cost-sharing to all Medicare beneficiaries residing in the service area of the MA plan. These benefits are offered by private company's that contract with Medicare to provide Part A and Part B benefits. May also be referred to as Medigap.	MA Plan or Medigap

Medicare Administrative Contractor	A private healthcare insurer that has been awarded a geographic jurisdiction to process Medicare Part A and Part B medical claims or DME claims for Medicare FFS beneficiaries. CMS relies on a network of MACs to serve as primary operational contact between Medicare and enrolled healthcare providers.	MAC
Medicare Learning Network	Series of articles that explain national Medicare policy in an easy to understand format. They focus on coverage, billing, and payment rules for specific provider types. Articles are prepared with assistance from clinicians, billing experts, and CMS subject matter experts.	MLN
Medicare Physician Fee Schedule	Listing of Medicare Part B covered services to healthcare providers which includes rates of reimbursement.	MPFS
Merit-based Incentive Payment System	This is a value-based program that was devised as part of the MACRA. In this program providers are assessed in a points-based manner on their quality, performance and cost. Their score directly imposes penalties or bonuses.	MIPS
Modifier	Indicate that a service or procedure performed has been altered by some specific circumstance, but not changed in its definition or code. They are used to add information or change the description of service in order to improve accuracy or specificity. Modifiers can be alphabetic, numeric or a combination of both, but will always be two digits.	
National Committee for Quality Assurance	Uses measurement, transparency and accountability to highlight top performers and drive improvement. The organization measures and then accredits health plans; and has grown to measure the quality of medical providers and practices. The organization provides the PCMH recognition as well as collects HEDIS data from health plans.	NCQA

National Correct Coding Initiative	Developed by CMS to promote national correct coding methodologies and to control improper coding leading to inappropriate payment in Part B claims. These coding policies are based on several resources including the AMA CPT® manual, national and local policies and edits, national societies, and analysis of standard medical and surgical practices. CMS annually updates these coding policies.	NCCI
National Coverage Determinations	Medicare coverage is limited to items and services that are reasonable and necessary for the diagnosis or treatment of an illness or injury (and within the scope of a Medicare benefit category). NCDs are made through an evidence-based process, with opportunities for public participation. In the absence of a national coverage policy, an item or service may be covered at the discretion of the Medicare contractors based on an LCD.	NCD
National Provider Identifier Entity Type I	A HIPAA compliant unique identification number for covered health care providers. Covered health care providers and all health plans and health care clearinghouses must use the NPIs in the administrative and financial transactions adopted under HIPAA. The NPI is a 10-position, intelligence-free numeric identifier (10-digit number).	NPI
National Plan and Provider Enumeration System	Database used for establishing and managing National Provider Identification numbers and related information and demographics.	NPPES
Net Collections	The amount a practice collects after adjustments are taken. A formula for calculating net collections is: Payment ÷ Charges x 100 = Net Collections.	

New Patient	A new patient is one who has not received any professional services (i.e., those face-to-face services rendered by physicians and other qualified health care professionals who may report evaluation and management services reported by a specific CPT® code from the physician/qualified health care professional or another physician/qualified health care professional of the exact same specialty and subspecialty who belongs to the same group practice, within the past three years.	
Non-payment	Instance in which a claim for healthcare services was not reimbursed by insurance plan to provider of care. A reason for the lack of reimbursement should be included in the remittance advice and corrective action by the provider's office should take place.	
Office of Civil Rights	Federal entity that regulates and enforces the Health Insurance Portability and Accountability Act (HIPAA).	OCR
Office of Inspector General, U.S. Department of Health and Human Services	Leader in efforts to fight waste, fraud and abuse in HHS programs, including Medicare and Medicaid. This entity has a nationwide network of audits, investigations and evaluations that is used for policy recommendations for decision-makers and the public. This network also assists in the development of cases for criminal, civil and administrative enforcement. The OIG develops and distributes resources to assist the healthcare industry in its efforts to comply with national fraud and abuse laws.	OIG
Organizational National Provider Identifier Type II	Health care providers who are organizations, including physician groups, hospitals, nursing homes, and the corporation formed when an individual incorporates him/herself. An individual who is a healthcare provider and who is incorporated, may need to obtain an NPI for themselves (Type 1) and an NPI for their corporation or LLC.	NPI

Originating Site	The location where a Medicare beneficiary gets physician or practitioner medical services through a telecommunications system. The beneficiary must go to the originating site for the services located in either: • A county outside an MSA • An HPSA in a rural census tract	
Out of Network	Not participating with an insurance plan which yields a different fee schedule or rate of reimbursement in comparison for in net work providers. This reimbursement rate might be favorable to the provider however based on the patients benefits and coverage; may also include a higher out of pocket expense for the patient.	OON
Out of pocket maximum	The maximum amount that a beneficiary or patient must pay for healthcare services under a qualified health plan before the health plan begins covering all services at 100%.	
Outpatient Prospective Payment System	The system that Medicare uses to determine its reimbursement to hospitals and mental health centers. CMS links this payment model to ASC payment systems.	OPPS
Panel	A listing of providers who are eligible and participating with an insurance plan. Services rendered by these providers will be covered and payable under a qualified beneficiaries benefits.	
Participation	Provider enrollment in a health plan that permits the in-network reimbursement for healthcare services for a qualified beneficiary.	
Patient Centered Medical Home	Model of care that puts the patients at the forefront of care to build better relationships between patients and their clinical care teams. This model includes standards and guidelines that must be met and followed by the healthcare provider which in turn will meet program requirements, accreditation and possible increased reimbursement.	PCMH

Patient Portal	A secure online platform that patients are given access to certain portions of their EHR. This platform is interfaced between the practice's EHR/PM software and the practice's website. Although features vary, many patient portals provide patients with the ability to send secure messages to the provider, schedule appointments, request refills, complete intake forms and pay for services.	
Patient Security Access Code	Used to protect the identity of a patient. Rather than using a patient's name, a code is used or given to others to identify a patient while maintaining their privacy.	PSAC
Patient Statement	A document that may distributed electronically or by paper to a patient or their guarantor that outlines dates and services provided, payments, adjustments and amount owed by the patient to a healthcare provider.	
Pay for Performance	CMS payment model to eligible providers of care, hospitals and other qualified healthcare providers that incentivizes quality over volume but introducing performance measures that must be met to qualify and receive incentive payments.	P4P
Pay to Address	The location in which an insurance plan will send reimbursement for approved healthcare services to the rendering provider. This location might be different from the practice location and should be confirmed during the credentialing and enrollment process.	
Payer of Last Resort	In the event that a patient is insured by State Medicaid and any other insurance, Medicaid is always the insurance to pay last.	

Payer Mix	Distribution of patient volume by the type of insurance being used to pay for healthcare services. This mix will indicate the quantity of payments received in the practice for each insurance type. This information can be used to trend reimbursement, denials and KPI's to manage the financial health of a practice.	
Payment Posting	The process of applying amounts paid for services rendered directly to patients accounts. The information for payment posting is usually derived from an EOB or an ERA. Accuracy in payment posting avoids credit balances and inaccurate patient and insurance balances.	
Place of Service	The location in which healthcare services were rendered to a patient by a qualified healthcare practitioner.	POS
Physician Quality Reporting System	Medicare program that connected provider reporting of healthcare quality data to provider reimbursement for services. It has been replaced within the QPP program's quality measures which serves as a percentage of the overall MIPS score.	PQRS
Physician Transaction Access Number	Medicare-only number issued to providers by MACs upon enrollment to Medicare. If the provider has relationships with one or more medical groups or practices or with multiple Medicare contractors, separate PTANS are generally assigned. Together, the NPI and PTAN identify the provider, or supplier in the Medicare program. CMS maintains both the NPI and PTAN in PECOS, the master provider and supplier enrollment system.	PTAN

Provider Enrollment, Chain and Ownership System	Online provider and supplier enrollment system used to submit Medicare enrollment applications, view, print and update enrollment information, complete enrollment revalidation process, withdraw voluntarily from the Medicare program and track Medicare enrollment applications.	PECOS
Point of Service Plan	Type of health insurance plan that is an HMO however it offers the beneficiary the flexibility to choose providers with limited to no referral form requirements. Most POS plans have increased service and supply coverage in comparison to an HMO plan.	POS
Practice Management Software	Allows for the automation of many day to day operations within a medical practice. Many PM systems may be interfaced with a clearinghouse and EHR system for interoperability. PM software and systems allow for electronic billing, scheduling, coding, and reporting. PM software and system features vary.	PM software or PM system
Pre-authorization/ Prior-authorization	Permission by an insurance plan for healthcare services or supplies. This permission is requested by the healthcare provider or healthcare organization prior to services or supplies being given. This approval will be included in claims submission for payment purposes.	
Pre-existing condition	A health problem that a patient had prior to insurance benefits being effective.	
Preferred Provider	A healthcare provider who has met certain criteria to be recognized by a health plan. Financial incentives may be given to patients for choosing this provider type and the provider may also obtain financial incentives from the health plan for meeting and maintaining certain criteria to be recognized as preferred.	

Preferred Provider Organization	An entity that pays for healthcare services to beneficiaries. Coverage within this type of organization provides greater flexibility than that of an HMO as well as expanded coverage. Most PPOs may not require a patient to obtain a referral to see a specialist.	PPO
Premium	The amount of money a subscriber must pay for health insurance coverage. For employer based health plans, this amount is withdrawn as a payroll deduction. This amount must be paid for health insurance coverage to remain active.	
Prescription Drug Monitoring Program	An electronic database that tracks controlled substance prescriptions in a state. PDMPs can provide health authorities timely information about prescribing and patient behaviors that contribute to the epidemic and facilitate a nimble and targeted response. This is a state-level intervention.	PDMP
Primary Care Physician	This healthcare provider is permitted and recognized to coordinate healthcare services as well as provide the first line of general healthcare services.	PCP
Primary Insurance	Health insurance plan and coverage that is responsible for paying for approved medical claims before another insurance in instances when a patient has more than one insurance.	
Prompt Payment Law	A group health plan, and a health insurance issuer offering health insurance coverage, shall provide for prompt payment of claims submitted for health care services or supplies furnished to a participant, beneficiary, or enrollee with respect to benefits covered by the plan or issuer, in a manner that is no less protective than the provisions of section 1842(c)(2) of the Social Security Act (42 U.S.C. 1395u(c)(2)).	

Protected Health Information	Information and data that can be linked back to identify a patient.	PHI
Provider	Healthcare professional who is accredited, certified or licensed to provide healthcare services. State laws govern individuals who are considered healthcare providers. These individuals are also referred to as Eligible Providers (EP).	EP
Qualified Independent Contractor	An entity that has a contract with the CMS to review appeals following a redetermination by a MAC and reconsiderations issued by Quality Improvement Organizations. QICs issue reconsiderations and represent level 2 of the Medicare appeals process.	QIC
Quality Improvement Organization	An entity that has a contract with CMS to monitor the appropriateness, effectiveness and quality of care furnished to Medicare beneficiaries. A QIO makes determinations as to whether the services provided were medically necessary and responds to beneficiary's complaints about the quality of care provided.	QIO
Qualified Medicare Beneficiary	Helps pay premiums, deductibles, coinsurance, and copayments for Part A, Part B, or both programs	QMB
Quality Payment Program	An incentive program mandated by the MACRA law for participating Medicare providers. The two program tracks are MIPS and APMs.	QPP
Quality and Resource Use Reports	Under the Value Modifier Program, QRURs provide information about the resources used and the quality of care furnished to a group's or solo practitioner's Medicare FFS beneficiaries. This report was no longer available after 2018.	QRUR

Reason Code   An explanation in the form of a standard code used by insurance plans to describe the purpose of a non-payment or denial. These codes are located on remittance advice and should be used by practice's to take corrective action to obtain reimbursement. Reason codes may be posted in Practice Management software for tracking purposes.

Reassignment   An individual physician or non-physician practitioner, except physician assistants, has granted a clinic or group practice the right to receive payment for the practitioner's services.

Reconsideration   The decision made in the second level of the Medicare appeals process. A reconsideration consists of an independent on-the-record review of an initial determination, including the redetermination and all issues related to payment of the claim. A reconsideration is conducted by a QIC or QIO under Medicare Parts A and B, by an Independent Review Entity or QIO under Part C, by an Independent Review Entity under Part D, and by the Social Security Administration for Medicare entitlement and certain premium appeals.

Redetermination   An independent review of an initial determination. A redetermination is conducted by the same Medicare contractor that issued the initial determination and refers to the decision made in the first level of the Medicare appeals process.

Recovery Audit Contractors	Identify and correct Medicare improper payments through the efficient detection and collection of overpayments made on claims of health care services provided to Medicare beneficiaries, and the identification of underpayments to providers so that the CMS can implement actions that will prevent future improper payments in all 50 states. These contractors conduct post-payment claims reviews.	RAC
Referral	The action of a referral is to transfer care from one provider to another. A referral form is provided by a primary care physician to a patient whose insurance plan requires prior approval to see a specialist or other approved ancillary service.	
Referring Provider	The provider who sends the patient to another provider. (i.e. PCP refers a patient to a specialist, in this situation the PCP is the referring provider). In the case of a consultation, the rendering provider must send a report back to the referring provider.	
Refund	Return of monies received, generally due to an overpayment. Each state and insurance participation contract has a timeframe in which monies should be paid or sent back from the date of identification of an overpayment.	
Registration	The process in which a healthcare practice obtains demographic, completion of forms, medical history, insurance information and payment in preparation for healthcare services. This information is entered into the patients medical records.	

Reimburse-ment	Payment for services rendered. This payment may come from sources such as insurance companies and patients. The amount paid may not be the complete amount that was charged for a service. If reimbursement is derived from an insurance company that a healthcare provider participates with, the reimbursement or amount paid will be the amount allowed by the insurance contract.	
Relative Value Unit	Measurement of the resources used by healthcare providers to provide services. Three factors included in this measurement are: (1) Physician Work (2) Practice Expense (3) Professional Liability Insurance Expense. CMS factors this into establishing payment for healthcare services.	RVU
Remittance Advice	This is a summary of services provided, payments made, non-payments or denials, adjustments allocated and patient responsibilities owed.	
Remittance Advice Remark Codes	RARCs are used to provide additional explanation for an adjustment already described by a CARC or to convey information about remittance processing. Each RARC identifies a specific message as shown in the Remittance Advice Remark Code List. There are two types of RARCs, supplemental and informational.	RARC
Resource-Based Relative Value Scale	The physician payment system used by the CMS and most other payers. Based on the principle that payments for physician services should vary with the resource costs for providing those services and is intended to improve and stabilize the payment system while providing physicians an avenue to continuously improve it.	RBRVS

Retraction	After an insurance plan has paid a claim; depending upon circumstances there is a decision to withdraw those funds back from the provider. This funds withdrawal may occur electronically on future payments. Reasons for retractions include but are not limited to incorrect or duplicate payment. Each state has time limits as to when retractions may occur which may be based on the original claim payment date or the date of service.	
Revenue Cycle Management	The management of the full breadth of cyclical activities which contribute to successful receipt of appropriate revenue in a timely manner.	RCM
Risk Adjustment	A method to offset the cost of providing health insurance for individuals—such as those with chronic health conditions—who represent a relatively high risk to insurers. Under risk adjustment, an insurer who enrolls a greater-than-average number of high-risk individuals receives compensation to make up for extra costs associated with those enrollees.	
Risk Adjustment Factor	Is based on health conditions a beneficiary may have as well as demographic factors. It is used to adjust capitated payments for beneficiaries enrolled in Medicare Advantage plans. The payments may vary based on a patients predicted level of risk or the cost to maintain that patients care.	RAF
Risk Management	Proactive approach to implementing processes, procedures and safeguards to minimize a practice's exposure to non-compliance of regulations and guidelines. This includes identifying and addressing vulnerabilities that create liabilities.	

RVS Update Committee	The RUC is a unique multispecialty committee dedicated to describing the resources required to provide physician services that the CMS considers in developing RVUs.	RUC
Secondary Insurance	An insurance plan that has been determined to pay insurance claims after a primary insurance plan. This conclusion has been made through a coordination of benefits determination.	
Self-Funded Plan	Type of plan usually present in larger companies where the employer itself collects premiums from enrollees and takes on the responsibility of paying employees' and dependents' medical claims. These employers can contract for insurance services such as enrollment, claims processing, and provider networks with a third party administrator, or they can be self-administered.	
Self-Pay	Payment arrangement in which the patient has no insurance or other external entity taking responsibility for payment of healthcare services. The patient or guarantor assumes full responsibility for all payments directly.	
Self-Referral	Occasion in which a provider has ownership in an entity in which they refer patients to that entity to obtain services or supplies and is reimbursed for those services or supplies. This practice is prohibited by the Stark Law.	
Sequencing Codes	Documenting CPT, ICD-10, and HCPCS codes based on level of severity.	
Sequestration	Mandatory reductions in Federal spending. These spending cuts impacted Medicare Part A and Part B payments for healthcare services and supplies.	

Sliding Fee Scale	Alternative healthcare cost structure based on a patient's ability to pay. These fees are a reduction to the practice's standard rates and applicable to patients who may have a financial hardship.
Social Security Act	An act to provide for the general welfare by establishing a system of Federal old-age benefits, and by enabling the several States to make more adequate provision for aged persons, blind persons, dependent and crippled children, maternal and child welfare, public health, and the administration of their unemployment compensation laws; to establish a Social Security Board; to raise revenue; and for other purposes. (Act of August 14, 1935) [H. R. 7260]
Specialist	Healthcare provider who focuses on a certain medical discipline. This provider focuses on managing, diagnosing and treating certain illnesses and symptoms. There is usually specialized training or board certification for this specialized area of medicine.
Stop Loss Provision	Applicable to some health insurance plans that have a deductible and a patient co-insurance responsibility. The provision is enacted after a certain amount is reached which then eliminates the beneficiary from paying further out of pocket or co-insurance expense. It established a maximum out of pocket expense.
Subscriber	The individual who is considered the primary account holder for insurance benefits. All other covered individuals on the same plan would be considered dependents of the subscriber

Substance Abuse and Mental Health Services Administration	Agency within the HHS that leads public health efforts to advance the behavioral health of the nation.	SAMHSA
Supplier	Defined in 42 CFR 400.202 and means a physician or other practitioner, or an entity other than a provider that furnishes health care services under Medicare.	
Sustainable Growth Rate	Formula used to determine the amount Medicare will pay providers for the services they provide. This formula includes factors such as growth in physician's cost, Medicare enrollments and GDP. The formula requires a reduction to physician Medicare payments when spending exceeds the SGR goal.	SGR
Tax Identification Number	The identifier assigned to an organization by the IRS for tax purposes. This is also an Employer Identification Number (EIN).	TIN
Telemedicine	The use of remote technology to provide diagnosis and treatment to patients.	
Tertiary Insurance	An insurance plan that has been determined to pay insurance claims after primary and insurance plans; they are considered the third insurance. This conclusion has been made through a coordination of benefits determination.	
Third-Party Administrator	An organization that insurance companies and self-funded plan outsource the administrative tasks related to and the processing of health insurance claims.	TPA

Time of Service Collections or Point of Service Collections	The process of requesting and obtaining payments from patients for services at the time those services are rendered. This process may occur during check in/registration or at check-out/discharge.	TOS or POS
Timely Filing	This is the window granted to submit a claim after the date-of-service. If a payer grants 60 days' timely filing, then claims must be submitted within 60 days of the date services were rendered.	
Transitional Care Management	The management of post-hospital-discharge patients for the 30 day period post-discharge with a face-to-face visit that occurs within two weeks of discharge. Primary purpose is to coordinate care for the patient, during their transition, to prevent readmission and/or condition exacerbation	TCM
Triple Aim (Now Quadruple Aim)	A concept to improve patient care, reduce healthcare costs and improve population health. A fourth aim has been introduced transforming to the Quadruple Aim which now includes Care team well-being with the goal of reduction of care team burn-out and improving the care team's experience.	
Unbundling	When codes that were previously grouped together for one payment are separated into their individual codes to allow for individual reimbursements by code instead of as a group.	
Uniform Consultation Referral Form	A form used by eligible Primary Care Physicians given to HMO, MCO, and patients whose health plans require a referral to specialists and other ancillary service providers. This form is given to meet referral requirements by insurance companies for billing applicable services.	UCRF

Uninsured Patient	A patient who is not covered by private, State or Federal health insurance coverage for healthcare services.	
Urgent Care Facility	Used to address condition, illnesses, and injuries that are serious enough to warrant immediate attention but may not have the severity to require a visit to an emergency room. Use of Urgent Care Facilities may reduce overcrowding and high costs of emergency rooms.	
Usual, Customary and Reasonable	The amount a health plan pays for covered medical services based on factors including geography and based on the charge amount providers charge for that or similar healthcare services.	UCR
Utilization Review	Process used to compare a patients healthcare status, care being provided with evidence-based criteria. This review process is thought to reduce over or improper utilization of resources thereby reducing waste.	UR
Value-Based Reimbursement	CMS payment model to eligible providers of care, hospitals and other qualified healthcare providers that incentivizes quality over volume but introducing performance measures that must be met to qualify and receive incentive payments.	
Virtual Group	Introduced through the MACRA legislation, CMS is attempting to reduce the burden of MIPS reporting for small physician practices. This provision allows practices with ten or fewer providers to work together in meeting MIPS requirements.	
Virtual Payment	A payment method used by some insurance companies instead of mailing paper checks to reimburse for healthcare services and supplies. There is a surcharge to the provider to process this payment type.	

Waste	Billing for unnecessary services to increase reimbursement without proper cause or patient benefit	Included in "FWA" as the W
Withhold Amount	A percentage of payment or set dollar amounts that are deducted from the payment to the physician group/physician that may or may not be returned depending on specific predetermined factors.	
Workers' Compensation	Disability compensation programs that provide wage replacement benefits, medical treatment, vocational rehabilitation and other benefits to certain workers or their dependents who experience work-related injury or occupational disease.	WC
W-9 Form	Form used during the credentialing and payer enrollment process by providers to authenticate a TIN, legal business name, address and federal tax classification. Practice's may choose to enter a pay to address on this form instead of a practice location for payment purposes.	

Index

NOTE: Page numbers in bold and italics refer to tables and figures.

About the Authors

Shawntea Moheiser, CMPE, CMOM

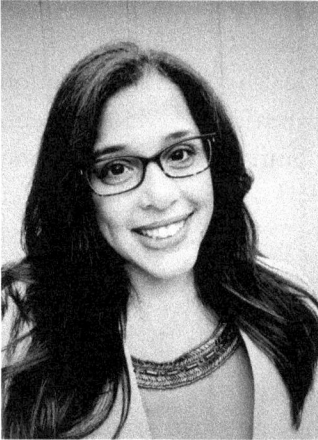

Shawntea (Taya) Moheiser is the owner of ITS Healthcare, LLC, a healthcare consulting company focused on innovation in healthcare management. Taya is the co-author of MGMA's 2019 publication "Revenue Cycle Management: Don't Get Lost in the Finance Maze", a contributing author to the Cleveland Clinic's 2018 publication "Voices of Innovation" and is a past speaker for national and state MGMA conferences. Taya has developed and implemented national care coordination programs, managed multi-specialty organizations, and provided executive leadership across the industry.

Taya is a current member of MGMA's Government Affairs Council, MGMA's Advocacy Team, and MGMA's E&M Workgroup. Additionally, she has served on various state and national associations related to the improvement of healthcare management. She is the current President-Elect for Nebraska HIMSS and has held several positions on state legislative committees focused on industry improvement.

Taya holds a bachelor's degree in Healthcare Management from Bellevue University and is currently seeking her master's degree in Healthcare Administration. Taya achieved CMPE status through MGMA and Certified Medical Office Management status through PMI.

457

In 2015, Taya was awarded the Governor's Volunteer Service Certificate from the State of Maryland based upon her efforts on the Maryland MGMA board and Maryland Physicians Association, MedChi. Taya's expertise is comprehensive throughout healthcare management with a special focus on revenue cycle management, operations compliance, and innovation in practice management. In her spare time she volunteers at Habitat for Humanity of Omaha, Omaha Lacrosse Club and Lauritzen Garden Guild.

Kem Tolliver, BS, CMPE, CPC, CMOM
President, Medical Revenue Cycle Specialists, LLC

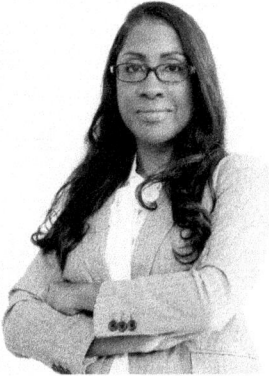

Kem holds dual Bachelor of Science degrees in Healthcare Administration and Organizational Management, graduating Summa Cum Laude and Magna Cum Laude, respectively. Her certifications include: Certified Medical Practice Executive (CMPE), Certified Professional Coder (CPC) and Certified Medical Office Manager (CMOM). For over 20 years, she has provided strategic and operational leadership to medical practices and hospitals. Kem is the President of Medical Revenue Cycle Specialists, LLC (MRCS). Medical practices she's managed have received MGMA˚ "Better Performing Practice" distinctions in the areas of Accounts Receivable and Collections. The MRCS team managed the start up of over 20 new medical practices in seven years.

In a desire to lead, Kem served on the Board of Directors of MD MGMA as the Chair of the Practice Management Committee, Chair of the Government Affairs Committee. She received MD MGMA's 2016 Outstanding Service Award and served as the 2018 State of Maryland ACMPE Representative.

Kem has provided testimony and guidance on healthcare legislation within the Maryland General Assembly. Kem served as a member of Maryland's 2018 General Assembly House of Delegates – Health & Government Operations Prior Authorization special session workgroup. Kem provides Maryland state-wide risk management training programs for Medical Mutual Insurance policy holders. She served as an Adjunct Professor of Revenue Cycle at Catonsville Community College.

From 2017-18, Kem served on the Board of Directors for Laurel Regional Hospital. She was a Mentor for the Prince George's County Public School's 2018 PTECH Health Innovation Program. Kem served on the Totally Linking Care-Maryland Interoperability Advisory Council and the Novitas JL Carrier Advisory Committee. She is the Co-Founder of Prince George's County Practice Manager's Association and was nominated by Nexus Health, Fort Washington Medical Center for the 2016 Community Health Award. Kem was awarded with the State of Maryland Governor's Volunteer Service Certificate for 2015-18.

www.ingramcontent.com/pod-product-compliance
Lightning Source LLC
Chambersburg PA
CBHW060425220326
41598CB00021BA/2295